The

Nutrition Hoax

BREAKFAST.

"If people let the government decide what foods they eat and what medicines they take, their bodies will soon be in as sorry a state as are the souls of those who live under tyranny."

— Thomas Jefferson

THE WICKEDNESS AND GREED OF THE PHARMACEUTICAL INDUSTRY:

A BILLION-DOLLAR BUSINESS

written by: Mr. Lemy

Preface

To New Beginnings.

First of all, thank you for picking up this book. It means a lot. Whether you're here out of curiosity, frustration with modern food choices, or a genuine desire to take control of your health, I want you to know that you're in the right place.

This book exposes the billion-dollar empires of the food industry, the government, Big Pharma, and the medical industry.

It enlightens and instructs readers about the meaning of nutrition and the true purpose of breakfast.

I wrote this book because, like many of you, I was once trapped in a cycle of misinformation about what to eat and what to avoid.

After digging into plenty of research, watching experts, and experimenting with different approaches to nutrition, I realized one thing: most of what we've been taught about food is wrong, and breakfast is a significant problem in today's world due to greed. It is causing way more damage than we're aware of.

A problem as "mere" as indoctrination about breakfast can set an entire population up for diseases such as–diabetes in the long run. The food industry thrives on confusion, illness, and misinformation.

The food you consume and how you consume it is harming you. You have been conditioned this way. The system isn't broken; **it's designed that way.**

Numerous videos on YouTube or X feature neurosurgeons, doctors, and other specialists in the "health" and medical fields admitting they have realized that they don't truly cure their patients

but rather hook them with a long-term solution that causes them to keep paying for treatments and medicaments without ever being cured until they die.

Do you really think this is about health and saving people?

Think about it for a sec, how many jokes and stories have you heard about people who find cures for diseases such as cancer, cures and solutions that could change the course of history but suddenly,

they decide to commit suicide and are later found lying on the floor with 23 gunshots wound on their back?

The 23 wounds may be exaggerated a little, but true stories inspire it, you know. If you believe the government genuinely seeks what is best for you, you may find this lecture challenging. **It's time to clarify the truth.**

Throughout my journey, I've been inspired by the work of experts, scientists, and health advocates who aren't afraid to challenge the status quo.

This guide results from countless hours of research, personal experience, and a passion for uncovering the truth about nutrition. My hope is that it will empower you to make informed choices and rethink everything you've been told about breakfast and nutrition in general.

This precious work is for those who are tired of feeling misled and ready to reclaim control over their bodies and health.

The same people who are giving you advice are the ones who thrive on you being ignorant and sick.

By the end of this book, you will have more knowledge about

food, digestion, weight loss, natural healing, nutrition, breakfast, bloating, and overall health than someone ever will by being a medical school student; hopefully, you won't be blinded by the lies anymore.

Let's run it.

"Breakfast is just a construct created by food companies. Many people do just fine without it, and skipping it may have numerous benefits."

- Dr. Micheal Mosley

(BBC Health Journalist and Author)

Genesis

Breakfast Begins.

"Breakfast is the most important meal of the day."

We've all heard that one before, right? But where does it originate? Is it true, or just another myth of science or lies from the government? Let's start by examining history.

Early Human Societies (Hunter-Gatherers)

No Set Breakfast:
Early humans didn't follow structured mealtimes. They ate whenever they had food, often fasting for extended periods until they found their next meal.

Morning Routine:
Instead of eating, they often began the day by hunting or gathering food. Fasting in the morning was a natural part of their lifestyle.

Ancient Civilizations (Egyptians, Greeks, Romans)

Egypt (c. 3000 BCE – 300 BCE):

Breakfast wasn't a formal meal but usually consisted of **bread, beer, onions, and fruit** if available.

Laborers and farmers might eat something simple before starting work, while wealthier individuals often skipped breakfast altogether.

Ancient Greece (c. 800 BCE – 146 BCE):

The Greeks had a light morning meal called **"akratisma,"** usually consisting of **barley bread dipped in wine, olives, or figs.**

It was more of a quick, practical snack rather than a sit-down meal.

Ancient Rome (c. 753 BCE – 476 CE):

Romans had a light morning meal called **"ientaculum,"** which consisted of **bread, cheese, and occasionally leftovers.** The elite often skipped breakfast, as it was considered unnecessary and indulgent.

The Middle Ages (5th – 15th Century)

Early Medieval Period:

Breakfast was viewed with suspicion, especially by the Catholic Church, which associated early eating with gluttony.

(Which oftentimes kind of is)

People who worked labor-intensive jobs (farmers, blacksmiths, etc.) often had a small meal at dawn, such as **bread, porridge, or ale.**

Late Middle Ages:

As cities grew and more structured work schedules developed, breakfast became more common.

Peasants and workers started eating morning meals regularly, consisting of **gruel, bread, and cheese.**

The wealthy still avoided breakfast, considering it unnecessary.

The Renaissance and Early Modern Period (15th – 18th Century)

Breakfast Gains Popularity:

As trade flourished and new foods became available (such as tea, coffee, and sugar), breakfast became more common.

In Europe, **bread with butter and ale or tea** became a typical morning meal, especially in England and France.

Coffeehouses and Social Change:

With the rise of coffeehouses in the 17th century, the idea of having a morning beverage alongside a light meal became more widespread among the upper class.

Pre-Industrial Revolution (18th – Early 19th Century)

More Regular Morning Eating Habits:

As urbanization increased, structured work hours in factories led to more people eating breakfast.

Typical working-class breakfasts included porridge, bread, eggs, and sometimes bacon. The upper class still preferred a late morning meal (brunch-like) consisting of lighter fare such as tea, pastries, and fruit.

Before the Industrial Revolution, breakfast was not a structured or heavily promoted meal. It was largely influenced by availability, social class, and work demands. **Most people either skipped it or had something simple and quick.**

The concept of breakfast as an "essential" meal didn't exist until it was popularized by businesses and the food industry in the 19th and 20th centuries.

Breakfast hasn't always been the structured, essential meal we know today. The way our ancestors lived was the right way. In order to feed you lies, they had to lie about our past.

"Who controls the past controls the future: who controls the present controls the past."

- George Orwell (1984)

They did that by telling us that our ancestors lived short, weak, miserable lives, were ignorant in many ways, and were unhealthy.

By telling you this nonsense, they created the opportunity to introduce you to a new health-wrecking lifestyle that would fill their pockets with jingly pieces of gold coins. One million dollars? That's pocket change for these people.

We are not evolving as a society. Society cannot evolve when it is founded on greed. The only reason more technology is being released to the public is for more control.

The more you depend on the system, the more they can control you. Most people know nothing about natural medicine.

Real medicine consists of herbs, plants, nature, the sun, and time. Not drugs.
These people are just legal drug dealers making billions, never curing you.

The fact that the average person has little to no knowledge about herbs, plants, and nature being the best healers is done on purpose.

If somebody thinks that society is evolving and that the ancient ways of living were inefficient, they will automatically accept the new ways and think of the ancient ways as "useless". We are just becoming more dependent on the system.

The idea of breakfast as a "must-have" meal is a relatively recent concept, largely shaped by industrialization, marketing, and the influence of the food industry.

As time goes on, society grows more gluttonous.
Fast forward to the Industrial Revolution, and breakfast began to take on new significance. With people working in factories for long hours, a morning meal became necessary to fuel their productivity.

During this time, breakfast foods like porridge and bread gained popularity as convenient options for the working class. However, it wasn't until the late 19th century that breakfast became truly commercialized.

James Caleb Jackson, a nutritionist and health reformer, is credited with creating the first manufactured breakfast cereal in 1863, which he named Granula.

Jackson developed this cereal by baking graham flour into brittle cakes, which were then crumbled and baked again. Due to its hardness, **Granula** required soaking in milk overnight before it could be eaten.

John Harvey Kellogg later improved James Caleb Jackson's initial cereal recipe, softened it, changed one letter, and brought **Granola** to the market. This began the omnipresent cereal empire as we know it today.

In 1917, dietitian Lenna F. Cooper wrote an article stating, **"Breakfast is the most important meal of the day."** The article was published in Good Health magazine, a publication associated with the Battle Creek Sanitarium **directed by John Harvey Kellogg.**

Their supposed health benefits were one of their first successful selling points. But in reality, eating cereals in the morning has little to no health benefits. Depending on what you eat.

This was all a hoax, *the breakfast hoax*. They crafted and propagated harmful false information to sell their products and prioritized money over the population's health.

In 1944, General Foods, the manufacturer of Grape-Nuts cereal, launched a marketing campaign titled "Eat a Good Breakfast—Do a Better Job." This campaign included advertisements claiming that "Nutrition experts say breakfast is the most important meal of the day," aiming to boost cereal sales during World War II.

Cereals' omnipresence results from years of persistent aggressive marketing and conditioning.
The cereal industry is currently putting it in the same league as American institutions such as the National Basketball Association (NBA) and gun stores, profiting billions by making people unhealthy and ignorant, two things you won't be after reading this book.

The idea that breakfast is the most important meal of the day originated from marketing rather than science.

In the early 20th century, cereal companies like Kellogg's **heavily promoted breakfast as essential**, emphasizing cereals as the go-to choice.

In reality, cereals are far from the go-to category, especially when eaten in the morning.

The cereal campaigns were designed to sell products, not to promote health. Don't eat those in the morning; if you have a choice, don't eat them at all.

After Kellogg's popularized cereals, other companies, such as Post, General Mills, and even fast-food chains like McDonald's and Tim Hortons, saw the potential for **massive profits by marketing breakfast** as an essential daily habit. They all took this golden opportunity to make money while destroying people's health and profiting from processed food and sugar cravings.

The phrase stuck, not because of scientific evidence, but because it was repeated in advertisements, schools (where kids get indoctrinated), and health publications. Over time, breakfast transformed from an optional meal into a societal norm and, for some, an addiction—one that food companies continue to capitalize on.

A granola bar that claims to be a 'healthy and energizing morning snack ' often contains **more sugar than a candy bar**.

The same goes for 'whole grain' cereals marketed as heart-healthy, which cause **massive blood sugar spikes.** And don't forget the McDonald's breakfast meals and the Tim Hortons donuts.

If they were really looking to heal people completely, they would have done it already.

They're filthy rich simply by feeding you lies (and cereals, in this case). The lies make you unhealthy; unhealthy people bring in the paycheck.

"Why won't the government do something about it?"
That's because they're in on it. It's not rocket science, you know.
It's a big club; you're not in it. You're the prey.

I am not saying that all doctors, surgeons, nurses, and others specializing in "health" and medicine are evil.

They are regular people who must pay the bills, just like you and me.

What I want you to know is that some of them, **most of them**, if not all, are doing the Devil's work without even knowing it.

When they eventually realize it, they often decide to quit their jobs. Others can't afford or don't have the guts to do so; therefore, they stay in their jobs and experience deep depression.

It's soul-wrenching to discover that years or even decades into your career, you've been prescribing people pills and treatments without ever really curing them. In other words, you've been unknowingly killing people for money.

If you think I'm talking nonsense with nothing to back it up, go watch the YouTube video:

"I Was An MIT Educated Neurosurgeon Now I'm Unemployed And Alone In The Mountains How Did I Get There?"

From the *Goobie and Doobie* channel. Thank me later.

Today, breakfast has become a billion-dollar industry dominated by processed, sugar-filled options. Cereal boxes crowd the shelves of supermarkets worldwide and are estimated to be a **10-billion-dollar industry annually.**

Money will always come before the population's health regarding what's important (for them). The only thing you can do about it is to change your ways.

Since childhood, you've been told that skipping breakfast will leave you weak, tired, and unable to focus. But have you ever wondered who benefits from this belief?
When will you start to look around you and see that the ones who can think for themselves and ask the real questions are the "weird ones"?

You go ahead and tell people that the government doesn't give one damn about its people, and they will label you as a "**conspiracy theorist.**" That's absurd, isn't it? The sheep are defending the very same wolves that are preying on them.

Our bodies are incredibly adaptable, and the need to eat immediately after waking up is nothing but a well-crafted marketing ploy.
"Breakfast kickstarts your metabolism" → FALSE.
Fasting naturally keeps metabolism high through fat oxidation and hormonal balance.

"You need breakfast to concentrate" → FALSE.
Mental clarity actually improves when fasting, as the body isn't digesting heavy meals.

"Skipping breakfast leads to weight gain" → FALSE.
Controlled eating windows improve insulin response and aid weight management.

"The idea that you must eat breakfast to maintain energy is completely outdated and misleading."

- Dr. Benjamin Bikman

(Metabolic Scientist)

"The notion that skipping breakfast leads to weight gain is based on flawed science. Metabolic flexibility is key."

- Dr. David Ludwig

(Harvard Nutrition Professor)

"Your body doesn't have a built-in clock that demands food at 7 AM. It needs fuel when it's ready, not when society says it should."

Keystone

Rise and Nourish.

Unless you want to regurgitate your guts like *Walter White on Breaking Bad*, I suggest you be wise about your first meal: **the breakfast.** I have a story to share about the one day I puked my guts out because I broke one of the most important rules of fasting.

Fasting has countless benefits that many people overlook. It's like a secret weapon for a long, healthy existence—especially when paired with regular exercise. Personally, I fast weekly, and not just any kind of fasting.

No, I go for the big leagues: **dry fasting**. No food, no water—it's intense, but I'm a seasoned pro, so it's become second nature to me.

On one of my usual weekly fasts, everything was smooth sailing. My mind was sharp, my focus was on point, and I cruised through the day like a fasting champion. Feeling a bit tired in the afternoon, I took a quick nap to recharge. When I woke up, it was time to break the fast. At this point, it was 5 p.m.—yes, breakfast at dinnertime.

Naturally, the first thing I reached for was water. Two tall glasses. Hydration is key, right? And let me tell you; after fasting, water tastes like the nectar of heaven.

But here's the thing about fasting: **it changes you**. Your hunger fades quickly; even small portions can feel like a feast.

After those two glasses, I was full and satisfied. I could've stopped there, but, well... **gluttony had other plans.**

Instead of listening to my body, I decided to *celebrate* breaking my fast. I dove straight into a **mountainous meal**: rice, eggs, sweet potatoes, macaroni salad, and two bananas. Oh, and I had donuts on standby for dessert because, you know, why not? Thankfully, divine intervention stopped me before I added those donuts to the chaos.

At first, all seemed well. I was living the post-fast dream. But then... it hit.

A few hours later, my stomach started staging a rebellion. I felt weak, hot, and uneasy. It was as if my body was screaming, "WHAT HAVE YOU DONE?!" And then the real punishment began: I vomited. Four times.

Not just any ordinary vomit, either—this was the kind of projectile regret that makes you reevaluate your life choices. If I'd eaten those donuts, I'm pretty sure my soul would have left my body.

After the ordeal, I collapsed into bed, completely drained, and prayed for better days.

Miraculously, by the next morning, I was back to normal, as if my body had forgiven me. Thank **God** for that!

When you're done fasting, **water often feels satisfying** because your body has adapted to operating in a state of deprivation, and your hunger cues are more nuanced and sensitive. When fasting (especially dry fasting), your body becomes dehydrated to some extent.

Thirst signals can be mistaken for hunger because the hypothalamus, the part of the brain that regulates both hunger and thirst, can confuse the two. Drinking water rehydrates you and alleviates the signals, making you feel like your hunger is satisfied.

During a fast, your stomach shrinks and slows down its activity.
Drinking water **fills your stomach**, stimulating stretch receptors that signal to your brain, "Hey, we're full!" This temporarily reduces the sensation of hunger.

Fasting lowers **ghrelin**, the "hunger hormone," while stabilizing insulin and blood sugar levels. By the time you finish fasting, your body has adjusted to operating without food, so hunger isn't as intense as you might expect. Water helps maintain this balance, tricking your body into thinking it's getting what it needs.

After fasting, your body enters a more mindful, sensitive state. Drinking water feels refreshing and fulfilling because your body is hyper-aware of anything entering your system. That's when it's most receptive to nutrients, including junk food. You've also trained your brain to be content with less, so simple things like water feel more satisfying.

When you finish fasting, your body isn't immediately craving food—it's prioritizing **hydration and gentle reentry.** Drinking water not only fulfills that immediate physiological need but also signals your brain that you're nourishing yourself, which can feel just as satisfying as eating.

This is why breaking a fast **slowly and with water or light foods, like bananas or mandarins,** is ideal. Your body is in a calm, efficient state, and jumping into heavy meals can overwhelm your system, causing you to question whether you are about to die or not, just like I did. You can actually use this "water fulfills hunger" effect to ease into eating mindfully and avoid overeating

Let this be a lesson to you; reading this

When breaking a fast, **less is more.** Don't let hunger (or the idea of hunger) fool you into eating a banquet. Start slow, keep it light, and listen to your body. Otherwise, you might find yourself in the same position I was—wondering if you'll survive another round of stomach warfare.

Vomiting after eating a heavy meal in the morning or after a fast is usually caused by overeating, just like I did.

Your stomach is simply overloaded with too much food, causing pressure and discomfort that can lead to nausea and vomiting as your body tries to relieve the pressure.

You may think it only happened because I went on a longer fast, but it can also happen to those who eat breakfast in the morning if they eat too heavy.

Do you know what a keystone is?

A **keystone** is the central stone in an arch that holds all the other stones in place. Without it, the entire structure would collapse. In a broader sense, it symbolizes something essential, foundational, and irreplaceable—what everything else depends on to stay intact.

Breakfast is like the keystone of our health and daily energy. It "holds everything together" by breaking the fast, replenishing the body, and setting the tone for how we function throughout the day.

The Real Meaning of Breakfast

The word "breakfast" literally means "breaking the fast," which is where its importance lies. After fasting, your body becomes more sensitive to nutrients and highly aware of what enters your system.

This is why **how you break your fast is as important as the fast itself.** If you consume processed junk or empty calories—like the sugary cereals or pastries that are often marketed as "breakfast foods"—you're doing your body more harm than good (harm only).

For example, I fasted for 24 hours, which was undoubtedly beneficial for my body. But because I broke my fast poorly—with a large, heavy meal instead of easing into it—I ended up vomiting everything I consumed. That experience taught me a crucial lesson: **breaking your fast the right way is key to reaping the full benefits of fasting.**

Breakfast Isn't About Morning

The phrase "Breakfast is the most important meal of the day" is partially true. However, people don't understand why it's true. Some say it's false, and others say it's true.

The idea that you must eat in the morning otherwise, you may be potentially harming yourself is completely false.

The importance lies not in the timing but in the **quality** of the meal. Breakfast doesn't have to be in the morning; it can happen any time you end your fast.

Eating in the morning is perfectly fine, but it's not mandatory for health. In the story I mentioned, I broke my fast at 5 p.m., which was my breakfast (break-fast).

For example, if your last meal is at 6 p.m., you sleep at 10, wake up at 7, and eat, you've just fasted 13 hours. If you eat at 6 p.m. instead, you just fasted 24 hours.

Your breakfast was at 6, although it wasn't in the morning. Fasting is the act of not eating, and it can still occur while you sleep. In fact, you can still benefit from fasting, even if most of it happens while you sleep.

Why Breakfast Is Key

Properly breaking your fast sets the foundation for your body's recovery and energy.

After fasting, your body is primed to absorb nutrients; what you give can either build or break you down.

What you eat first will set your body and dictate its energy for the rest of the day. The key is to consume nourishing, whole foods that support your system—not processed garbage disguised as "convenience."

In short, **breakfast is the keystone of your health,** but it's not about the time on the clock—it's about what you're feeding your body when it's ready to break the fast.

The focus should be on quality, balance, and intention. Done right, breakfast reinforces the benefits of fasting and fuels your day, no matter what time you choose to eat. Don't eat too late, of course. A healthy man has a thousand desires, a sick man only has one.

When you delay eating in the morning, your insulin levels remain low, allowing your body to continue using **stored fat for energy** instead of relying on incoming food.

You're wondering why food companies and governments lie so much?

That's because most people can't think for themselves.

If you have a healthy brain, you can connect the dots and realize that skipping breakfast will not make you gain weight, it literally burns fat. It's a dumb lie based on fear and marketing. How can you fall for that?

Did you know that some of the most famous studies claiming **'breakfast is essential for weight loss'** were funded by the very companies selling breakfast products?

Science should be impartial, but money often speaks louder than the truth.

Skipping eating in the morning is beneficial; it burns fat. Don't worry if you're a gym bro; you won't lose your hard-earned muscle mass.

As a matter of fact, fasting increases human growth hormone significantly.

When you fast, your insulin levels drop. Insulin and HGH are inversely related—low insulin creates an environment where HGH production can skyrocket. Studies show that fasting can increase HGH levels by as much as **300–2000%**, depending on the duration.

Preserves Lean Muscle Mass:
HGH plays a key role in maintaining and building muscle. During fasting, your body uses HGH to protect your muscles from being broken down for energy while promoting fat burning instead.

Improves Fat Burning:
HGH stimulates lipolysis, which is the breakdown of fat for energy. Fasting enhances this process by making your body more reliant on fat stores, which helps with body recomposition (burning fat while preserving or building muscle).

Supports Testosterone Production:
HGH works synergistically with testosterone. Both hormones play essential roles in muscle growth, recovery, and overall vitality. It enhances factors (like lower insulin and body fat levels) that support optimal testosterone production.

Burn fat, Build muscle.

Here are some credible references if you want to do some research

Healthline, National Library of Medicine (PubMed), Nature, Endocrinology and Metabolism Journal

Fasting promotes **ketosis**, a state in which the body burns fat more efficiently for fuel.
It also increases **lipolysis** (a metabolic process that breaks down fat stores into energy for the body) and the breakdown of fat cells.

Not eating in the morning prolongs your fast and keeps the fat-burning mechanism on the clock. Again, breakfast literally means "breaking the fast"—it has nothing to do with eating when you wake up.

Eating when you wake up is not wrong or harmful, as long as you break your fast in a nutrient-dense way.

The problem is that most people eat in the morning because they've been told it's harmful and bad not to. Sometimes, they're not even hungry; they just do it for the culture.

If this is you, you deserve to know there are countless benefits to not eating several hours after you have woken up and doing something such as taking a walk or doing intense exercise instead. No, you won't die if you exercise on an empty stomach, relax.

But think about it; if your body is more receptive and sensitive to nutrients after a fast: Why would anyone break their fast and fill it with a **chunk of sugar and refined carbohydrates, such as cereals?**

Why would they encourage you to do so?

If your body is sensitive to the foods you consume after a fast, nourishing it with healthy options like eggs, meat, fruits, and vegetables is the only option. Aim to provide a nutrient-dense meal. If this seems too heavy to eat in the morning, remember that breakfast is not strictly about the time of day; instead, it's about the nourishment of the meal. Feel free to experience it yourself.

Picture this:

one morning, you wake up and reach for a bowl of sugary cereal, something that's been marketed as the perfect start to your day.

You eat and feel a quick energy spike, but within an hour or two, notice the crash. Your hunger creeps back far too quickly, and you're left sluggish, craving more food or, even worse— another sugary snack.

Now, pay attention to how your body responds. Are you satisfied? Energized? Or do you feel drained and stuck in a hunger and low energy cycle?

Now, let's try a different approach the next day. When you wake up, skip the sugary start and hydrate instead.

Take a glass of water, add a squeeze of fresh lemon juice, and a pinch of sea salt or Himalayan salt. This combination gives your body a boost of electrolytes, ensuring efficient hydration and setting the tone for your day. Avoid table salt, as it's often stripped of its minerals.

For the next five hours, refrain from eating anything. Use this time to focus, be productive, and prepare yourself mentally and physically for what's ahead.

During this fasted state, head out and exercise. Whether it's cardio, a brisk walk, weightlifting, or some calisthenics, push yourself in a way that challenges your body.

You'll notice something powerful—your body feels sharper, lighter, and more capable than it does when weighed down by an early, carb-heavy meal.

When the time comes to break your fast, do so intentionally. Forget the processed junk or sugar-loaded meals.

Instead, nourish your body with **real food**: eggs, avocados, meat, sweet potatoes, fruits—simple, wholesome ingredients that fuel you.

Start with something light if you need to, like a bowl of fresh fruits, and follow up with a bigger, more substantial meal later in the day.

Your body will thank you for this balance of nutrients and sustained energy.

Why This Works

You'll notice that the second approach does something remarkable: it gives you **energy, focus, and discipline** throughout the day.

You'll feel fuller for longer, and instead of being a slave to cravings or hunger spikes, you'll find yourself in control. If you commit to this pattern for 10 days, the changes will become evident—you'll feel lighter, stronger, and more mentally sharp.

Keep this up for 30 days, and the benefits will multiply. Not only will your body adapt to this new rhythm, but you'll also develop a sense of discipline and self-control that spills over into every area of your life. You'll move with purpose and intention, no longer at the mercy of sugary highs and crashing lows. Gluttony can really mess up your life more than you're aware of.

The Flexibility of Breakfast

Let's put to rest the myth that breakfast has to happen at a specific time. Maybe you wake up at 7 AM, fast for five hours, exercise, and have your first meal—your **breakfast**—at noon.

Someone else, like Robert, might eat at 8 AM, while Kyle's first meal might not happen until 3 or 4 PM. That's okay.

Your breakfast timing doesn't matter if you don't eat too late. What matters is **what you eat, how you break your fast, and your consistency.**

Your schedule and goals will vary, but don't let a busy life become an excuse for poor discipline. Fasting and intentional eating benefit those prioritizing their health and pushing past fleeting desires.

Insulin Spikes and Crashes

Mastering your insulin response is like finding the key to stable energy, clear thinking, and metabolic health.

It's not about eliminating carbs—it's about choosing the right kinds and managing your meals in a way that keeps your body balanced. It's part of why your fasting routine, when paired with smart refeeding practices, is so powerful for long-term health.

Managing insulin levels is crucial for maintaining **stable energy, preventing chronic diseases, and supporting overall health.**

Avoiding foods that cause rapid insulin spikes and focusing on balanced, nutrient-dense meals can lead to long-term health benefits, increased energy, and a reduced risk of metabolic disorders. By controlling your insulin responses, you can control your health.

"We made bacon and eggs a thing. We convinced the public that breakfast had to be heavy to be healthy."

- Edwards Bernays

(Father of Public Relations, referring to breakfast marketing)

"Skipping breakfast and extending the fasting period can actually improve metabolism and brain function rather than hinder them."

- Dr. Mark Mattson

(Neuroscientist, National Institute on Aging)

Why Eating Too Late Can Harm Your Body

Eating too late, especially close to bedtime, disrupts digestion, metabolism, and overall health in ways most people don't realize. Eating too late makes the body less efficient at breaking down food. Digestive activity slows down as the body prepares for rest.

Your body uses energy to repair, detox, and regulate hormones during sleep. However, forcing it to digest food can lead to issues like indigestion, bloating, and acid reflux—that uncomfortable burning sensation in your chest or throat.

Another common consequence is diarrhea or stomach pain. When the digestive system is rushed and overloaded, it leads to improper nutrient absorption and irritation in the gut.

Even if you don't feel immediate symptoms, eating late still negatively affects your body. It disrupts insulin regulation, increases fat storage, and weakens gut health.

Over time, this pattern can lead to weight gain, poor sleep quality, and even long-term metabolic issues like insulin resistance and inflammation.

Just because you don't feel bad after eating late doesn't mean it isn't harming you. The damage happens silently, affecting digestion, slowing metabolism, and interfering with your body's natural healing process.

If you want to wake up feeling lighter, more energized, and with a stronger gut, eating earlier is best to allow your body the time it needs to digest before sleeping fully.

How Many Hours Before Sleep Should You Stop Eating?

To optimize digestion, metabolism, and sleep quality, avoid eating for 3 to 4 hours before bedtime.

The Best Timing for Your Last Meal

At least 3–4 hours before sleep (Ideal)
At least 2 hours before sleep (Okay, but not optimal)
Less than 2 hours before sleep (Risk of indigestion, acid reflux, and poor sleep)

What If You Feel Hungry Before Bed?

If you must eat, opt for light, easy-to-digest foods like:
Herbal tea
A small handful of nuts
A piece of fruit (but avoid sugar-heavy ones)

Going to Bed Hungry: A Shortcut to Fat Burning & Metabolic Reset

If you're serious about **fat loss, digestion, and metabolic health, going to bed on an empty stomach** can work in your favor.

When you stop eating early and **sleep in a fasted state**, your body doesn't have to focus on digestion. Instead, it shifts into **repair mode, fat-burning, and deep detoxification.**

Here's Why Sleeping Hungry Can Be Beneficial:

Initiates Fat Burning Earlier – Since insulin levels stay low, your body starts tapping into stored fat for energy instead of glucose.

Increases Growth Hormone (GH) Production – GH helps **burn fat, build muscle, and repair tissues**—and it's highest during deep sleep when you're fasting.

Improves Digestion—Overnight, your gut gets a full **reset,** leading to **better bowel movements and less bloating** in the morning.

Enhances Sleep Quality—Contrary to popular belief, **going to bed hungry can help you fall into deeper, more restorative sleep.**

Boosts Longevity – Fasting before sleep reduces inflammation, supports cellular repair (autophagy), and improves insulin sensitivity.

People panic at the idea of skipping a meal before bed, but **the truth is, your body doesn't need food 24/7.** If anything, late-night eating does more harm than good. Most people eat at night out of **habit, boredom, or cravings**, not actual hunger.

Take control. Let hunger work in your favor. By sleeping on an empty stomach, you'll wake up **leaner, lighter, and more energized**—while your body burns fat like a machine overnight.

When you're working out and you have to push yourself, it burns; it's painful and doesn't feel good.

But you know it was worth it when you see the results, the growth, the pump, the energy boosts, the health benefits, and the mindset change.

Always Remember, **Discipline Over Gluttony.** Purpose **Over Pleasure.**

The Danger of Insulin Spikes and Crashes

Insulin is a hormone produced by the pancreas that helps regulate blood sugar levels by allowing glucose to enter cells for energy or storage. While insulin is essential for normal bodily function, **frequent spikes and crashes** can have detrimental effects on health.

What Causes Insulin Spikes?

Refined Carbohydrates and Sugars: Foods like white bread, pastries, sugary cereals, sodas, and candies cause rapid increases in blood sugar. Does this sound familiar?

These are foods people break their fasts with.

They have been pushed to do so.

Overeating: Consuming large quantities of food, especially processed carbs, forces your pancreas to produce more insulin.

Lack of Fiber: Fiber slows down glucose absorption. Low-fiber foods lead to quicker insulin responses.

The Cycle of Spikes and Crashes

Insulin Spike: Blood sugar levels soar after consuming a high-sugar or high-carb meal. In response, the pancreas releases a surge of insulin.

Rapid Glucose Uptake: Insulin quickly moves glucose into cells, causing blood sugar levels to drop sharply.

Crash: A sudden drop in blood sugar can cause feelings of fatigue, irritability, and hunger and often prompt further unhealthy eating.

Repeat Cycle: Frequent repetition of this cycle can lead to metabolic disorders over time.

Health Risks of Insulin Spikes and Crashes

Increased Fat Storage:

Insulin promotes the storage of excess glucose as fat, leading to weight gain and difficulty in losing weight.

Insulin Resistance:

Over time, cells become less responsive to insulin, forcing the pancreas to produce more. This can lead to **type 2 diabetes**, where the body struggles to regulate blood sugar effectively.

(Note)

The information in this book is not meant for you just to read. You must study it. Do that and you'll gain real knowledge about nutrition, fasting, health, longevity, and disease prevention. You'll know more about nutrition than doctors learn in Med School.

Energy and Mood Swings:

Insulin crashes cause fatigue, brain fog, irritability, and cravings for more sugar, perpetuating unhealthy eating habits.

Increased Risk of Chronic Diseases:

Chronic high insulin levels are associated with heart disease, obesity, hypertension, and certain cancers.

Hormonal Imbalances:

Elevated insulin can disrupt other hormones like testosterone and estrogen, affecting mood, libido, and fertility.

Accelerated Aging:

Frequent insulin spikes increase oxidative stress and inflammation, contributing to the aging process and age-related diseases.

These are the 56 **most common names** for sugar.

Agave nectar

Barbados sugar

Barley malt

Beet sugar

Blackstrap molasses

Brown rice syrup

Brown sugar

Buttered syrup

Cane juice crystals

Cane sugar

Caramel

Carob syrup

Castor sugar

Confectioner's sugar

Corn syrup

Corn syrup solids

Crystalline Fructose

Date sugar

Demerara sugar

Dextran

Dextrose

Diastatic malt

Diastase

Ethyl maltol

Evaporated cane juice

Florida crystals

Fructose

Fruit juice

Fruit juice concentrate

Galactose

Glucose

Glucose solids

Golden sugar

Golden syrup

Grape sugar

High-fructose corn syrup

Honey

Icing sugar

Invert sugar

Lactose

Malt syrup

Maltose

Maple syrup

Molasses

Muscovado sugar

Organic raw sugar

Panocha

Raw sugar

Refiner's syrup

Rice syrup

Sorghum syrup

Sucrose

Treacle

Turbinado sugar

Yellow sugar

Syrup

Some of these sugar alternatives can act worse than plain sugar when it comes to their effects on the body. Here's why:

High-Fructose Corn Syrup (HFCS)

Why it's worse: HFCS is highly processed and contains a higher ratio of fructose than regular sugar. Excessive fructose is linked to insulin resistance, increased fat storage (especially around the liver), and higher risks of metabolic syndrome.

Commonly found in: Sodas, candy, baked goods, and processed snacks. **Sometimes in morning foods.**

Agave Syrup/Nectar

Why it's worse: Agave syrup is marketed as a "healthy" sugar alternative but can contain up to 90% fructose. That's even higher than HFCS! Overconsumption of fructose is associated with liver damage, fat gain, and inflammation.

Commonly found in: "Natural" or "organic" labeled snacks, desserts, and drinks.

Maltose and Malt Syrup

Why it's worse: These are high on the glycemic index (GI), meaning they cause rapid blood sugar and insulin spikes. This leads to crashes and cravings and, over time, can contribute to insulin resistance.

Commonly found in: Cereals, candies, and processed foods. **Again, morning foods.**

Evaporated Cane Juice

Why it's worse: It sounds fancy and "natural," but it's essentially the same as regular table sugar. It's just a marketing term to disguise sugar in a "healthier" light.

Commonly found in: "Healthy" granola bars, yogurts, and baked goods. **Things people eat in the morning.**

Fruit Juice Concentrate

Why it's worse: Stripped of fiber, these concentrates act as pure sugar in the body, leading to insulin spikes. The fructose content is also high, which can overburden the liver and lead to fat accumulation.

Commonly found in: Fruit-flavored drinks, "natural" candies, and even baby food.

Dextrose and Glucose

Why it's worse: These are simple sugars with an extremely high glycemic index. They cause immediate blood sugar spikes and crashes, promoting cravings and contributing to poor energy regulation.

Commonly found in: Energy drinks, processed snacks, and baked goods.

Why They're Worse

Many of these sugars are more processed than plain table sugar, removing any potential natural benefits (like trace minerals or fiber).

Their high fructose content or rapid absorption can damage insulin levels, liver function, and overall metabolic health.

Companies often use these alternatives to make food seem healthier by avoiding "sugar" on the ingredient list.

The Takeaway

While plain sugar isn't "good," these alternatives can often be worse because of their metabolic effects or how they're marketed to mislead consumers.

The best approach is to minimize processed sugars entirely and focus on natural, whole-food sources like fruits (in moderation) or natural sweeteners like raw honey or pure maple syrup.

You will often see **"no added sugar"** on labels, but there may be ingredients that act worse than sugar.

Manufacturers often replace sugar with other substances, like **corn starch** or sugar alternatives, that still spike blood sugar, trigger insulin responses, and contribute to long-term health issues. It's just a marketing trick, you know.

"No added sugar" only refers to table sugar (sucrose) or similar sweeteners directly added to the product.

Ingredients like **fruit juice concentrate, maltodextrin, dextrose, or corn syrup solids** can still be added without breaking the "no added sugar" claim.

These ingredients act worse than sugar in the body, spiking blood glucose levels and triggering the same harmful effects as refined sugar. People think that because there's **"no added sugar,"** it's a healthier alternative. Meanwhile, it could be worse than a product with added sugar. Do you see how bad you're being played right now?

It also happens with corn starch.

Corn starch can act worse than sugar in some ways, depending on how it's processed and consumed.

Breakdown into Glucose:
Corn starch is made up of long chains of glucose molecules (a polysaccharide). Once consumed, your body rapidly breaks it into glucose, spiking blood sugar levels almost as quickly as eating plain sugar.

High Glycemic Index (GI):
Corn starch has a **higher glycemic index** than table sugar.
For example:

Table sugar (sucrose): GI ~65

Corn starch: GI ~85-95
This means corn starch causes a **faster and sharper blood sugar spike**, which leads to stronger insulin surges and subsequent crashes.

Overuse in Processed Foods:
Corn starch is a cheap, flavorless thickener used in processed foods. It doesn't add sweetness but still contributes to blood sugar imbalances. It's commonly found in:

Sauces, gravies, soups

"No sugar added" baked goods

Gluten-free foods (as a replacement for wheat)

Hidden in Ingredients like Maltodextrin:

Maltodextrin is a processed form of corn starch with an even **higher glycemic index** than corn starch itself (GI ~110). It's often added to products to bulk them up, act as a stabilizer, or replace sugar while still having the same harmful effects.

Why Corn Starch Can Be Worse Than Sugar

Sugar contains **fructose** and **glucose.** While fructose has its own problems (liver overload, fat storage), the glucose in sugar is slower to metabolize than the rapidly absorbed glucose from corn starch.

Corn starch offers **no sweetness or flavor**, so it's "invisible," making people unaware of its impact.

Its overuse in processed foods means you can unknowingly consume large amounts, leading to chronic insulin spikes, weight gain, and insulin resistance.

This aims to illustrate just how much our food has been processed. The situation is so severe that much of it can't even be classified as real food.

Additionally, they (Big Pharma, advertisements you see, and Food companies) have claimed that these processed snacks and baked goods are a go-to and ideal choice for breakfast. Meanwhile, it's killing you.

Remember, when you eat in the morning, you're coming out of a fast, so why would they tell people to eat such destructive foods and processed snacks, especially when your body is hyper-aware and receptive to nutrients?

You're setting yourself up for a **big old diabetes 2.** You're investing your money in long-term suicide stocks. Best believe me when I say this: **it's a blue-chip stock.**

If you're drowning your system in sugary drinks, processed snacks, and refined carbs every day, even worse as a breakfast, you're on the express train to insulin-resistance ville. Type 2 diabetes doesn't show up overnight—it's a slow buildup caused by years of dietary abuse.

Sometimes people don't eat in the morning thinking they have skipped breakfast, then, they will go eat Mcdonald's as their first meal of the day.

It's still breakfast. It's breakfast, but a really health-destroying one. Eating fast food as a breakfast is probably the worst thing you could do, especially if it's McDonald's.

How to Step Off the Diabetes Train

Quit the Sugar Habit: Cut out sugary sodas, cereals, and snacks—these are your biggest enemies.

Sugar is one of the biggest addictions out there and also one of the biggest pre-aging factors.

Balance Your Meals: Pair healthy carbs with protein and fats to stabilize blood sugar.

Move Your Body: Exercise improves insulin sensitivity, so get moving. Walk, lift weights, or do anything that gets your blood flowing.

Exercise is mainly known as one of the causes of a long and healthy life.

Hydrate Smartly: Swap sugary drinks for water, herbal teas, or electrolyte-rich beverages (hold the sugar).

A single 7Up can (or similar sugary soda) often contains **around 40 grams of sugar**, exceeding the **recommended daily limit** for adult males **(36 g)**. For women, it's nearly **double their daily limit (25 g)**. Some kids gulp down two of these in a day. That's how bad the situation is. (The sugar from the whole foods doesn't count)

Eat Whole Foods: Stick to foods in their natural state—
vegetables, proteins, healthy fats, and fruits in moderation.

Regularly exceeding these limits contributes to insulin
resistance, weight gain, and chronic diseases like type 2
diabetes and heart disease.

**Why are processed foods, seed oils, and sugar promoted
so much if they're so deadly?**

It's because of...

Wickedness

A patient cured is a customer lost.

A business needs customers to work because customers are
the source of revenue that allows a company to operate and
generate profit; without customers purchasing goods or
services, a business cannot sustain itself; essentially,
customers are the lifeblood of any business.

Now, if you haven't watched the video I recommended earlier in this book,

"I Was An MIT Educated Neurosurgeon Now I'm Unemployed And Alone In The Mountains How Did I Get There?"

from the **Goobie and Doobie** channel, on YouTube, I recommend you do.

The video highlights a neurosurgeon who realized that his spine surgeries weren't effectively addressing the root causes of his patients' problems.

Although his surgeries provided temporary relief—often lasting around six months—patients frequently returned with the same issues, sometimes even after he performed what he believed were flawless procedures.

This recurring cycle prompted him to reassess his approach. He observed that patients who maintained a healthy lifestyle, including nutritious diets, adequate sleep, regular exercise, strong social connections, and a focus on both physical and mental well-being, experienced significantly better health outcomes.

The neurosurgeon understood that true healing goes beyond surgical intervention, emphasizing the importance of overall lifestyle choices in achieving long-term health. The problem is that patients weren't really aware of that. They really relied on the system.

When you do these things, your body heals. However, he later acknowledged that hospitals need money, which they earn by charging people for temporary solutions (like surgery). These solutions provide short-term relief from pain and make problems seem to disappear for a while, but they tend to resurface.

If they found a way to make people healthy and couldn't charge them for it **(lifestyle choices, nutrition, and mental health)**, they would be left with nothing. This boils down to one thing: the goal isn't to cure people; the goal is to provide them with solutions to ensure they keep coming back, and every time they come back, they pay.
You become a loyal customer.

This is why you often see people with certain diseases taking medication regularly. Unfortunately, this cycle never ends; they are always taking pills, and often, the dosage never stops increasing. This leaves patients with no choice but to purchase larger amounts of their medications, which inevitably costs more money—money that goes to, you know who. **Patients are customers. Cure one patient, and you just lost a customer.**

A patient cured is a lost customer.

How much is your health worth? Do you want to let yourself turn into a walking ATM in the eyes of the medical industry?

As mentioned earlier, cereal companies funded "scientific" studies claiming that eating in the morning was so important that people needed to eat cereals in the morning.

You can't base your health choices on all scientific research because many scientists will just agree with whoever puts money in their pockets.

The ones that don't agree get silenced. Money speaks louder than the truth. Eating sugary foods, empty calories, and refined carbs kills you in the long run, but that's not what they tell you. Do you see how far they were willing to go to make money?

They prioritize profit over health. Over time, the idea that you must eat something—anything—first thing in the morning became a widespread belief.

This mindset led many to consume junk food and sugary cereals in the morning, ultimately benefiting cereal companies. Scientists also profited from promoting these ideas. Everyone won except for those who got sicker and gained weight. Meanwhile, the medical industry continues to reap billions from these consequences yearly.

A significant contributor to the prevalence of type 2 diabetes is the consumption of sugary breakfast foods. Regular intake of processed cereals and pastries leads to rapid spikes in blood sugar levels, increasing the risk of developing insulin resistance over time.

Studies have shown that diets high in ultra-processed foods are linked to weight gain and a higher risk of chronic conditions such as diabetes. Do you see how all this correlates to promoting processed foods for breakfast?

This correlation between diet and disease underscores concerns about the medical industry's financial incentives. The substantial profits derived from diabetes treatments may contribute to a lack of emphasis on preventive measures and public education about the risks associated with high-sugar diets.

Breaking Down the Diabetes Industry's Profits:

The medical industry thrives on **managing** chronic diseases rather than curing them. Here's how:

Diabetes is a Lifelong Condition for Most Patients

Type 2 diabetes is largely **preventable and reversible** through diet and lifestyle changes.

However, **the medical system focuses on symptom management rather than prevention or reversal**—keeping patients dependent on medication.

Big Pharma and Diabetes Drugs

The pharmaceutical industry generates **billions** selling insulin, metformin, and other diabetes medications.

Example: The global diabetes drug market was valued at over **$60 billion in 2023** and is expected to grow.

Insulin prices have skyrocketed, even though it has existed for over a century.

Hospital Visits and Complications

Diabetes leads to **serious complications** like kidney failure, blindness, and amputations—leading to **more medical expenses**.

Dialysis, a treatment for kidney failure (often caused by diabetes), is a **multi-billion-dollar industry** alone.

Why They Push Unhealthy Diets

The food industry profits from selling cheap, high-sugar, highly processed foods.

These foods cause metabolic issues, leading to diabetes, which in turn **feeds the medical industry**.

Isn't it crazy how people are encouraged to eat sugar in the morning? Especially with the fact that you are coming out of a fast and sugar is one of the worst things to eat after a fast, but it's the most pushed thing for morning foods. Why? Because it's the most destructive.

It's a cycle: Processed food → Disease → Expensive Treatment → Lifelong Medical Dependency (loyal customer).

The Real Issue: Profit Over Prevention

If diabetes was truly cured at scale, **Big Pharma, hospitals, and insurance companies would lose billions** in recurring revenue.

Instead of educating people on real solutions (whole foods, fasting, and insulin control), they push **medication as the only answer.**

This explains why **misleading dietary advice**—like "breakfast cereals are healthy"—is still promoted and popular.

Here are some credible sources if you want to do some research.

American Diabetes Association (ADA), Verywell Health, Harvard T.H. Chan School of Public Health

In other words, **you have no future if you blindly follow advice from the same liars who profit from your unhealthiness.**

Unless it's directly related to the condition you're being treated for, notice how nutrition and lifestyle are often really overlooked when you go to the doctor. Doctors receive little to no education in nutrition.

In 2017, poor dietary habits were linked to approximately 11 million deaths worldwide, accounting for about 22% of all adult fatalities. The majority of these deaths were due to cardiovascular diseases, followed by cancers and type 2 diabetes.

As of 2025, this trend has continued to worsen **annually**. The World Health Organization (WHO) reports that noncommunicable diseases (NCDs), such as heart disease, stroke, type 2 diabetes, and certain cancers, are responsible for 75% of non-pandemic-related deaths globally.

The WHO emphasizes that up to 80% of heart disease, stroke, and type 2 diabetes cases, as well as 40% of cancers, could be prevented by improving diet, increasing physical activity, and avoiding harmful habits like smoking and excessive alcohol consumption.

Poor nutrition often leads to chronic inflammation, which is a key factor in many diseases, including arthritis, autoimmune disorders, and neurological conditions like Alzheimer's disease. Diets high in processed sugars, refined carbohydrates, and unhealthy fats contribute to systemic inflammation. Additionally, an unhealthy diet can harm the gut microbiome, which is critical to immunity, digestion, and mental health. A compromised gut can lead to issues like autoimmune diseases, allergies, and even depression.

It's concerning that despite nutrition's significant role in disease prevention and development, many healthcare professionals receive minimal education on this topic. This gap underscores the need for greater emphasis on nutrition in medical training and public health initiatives.

If you want to reference the sources (Data from the World Health Organization, 2025)(Sources: WHO, CDC, NCBI)

When you visit the doctor, what do they usually ask?

"What brings you in today?"

"Have you had any previous illnesses or surgeries?"

"Do any diseases run in your family?"

"Are you taking any medications or supplements?"

"Do you smoke or drink alcohol?"

"How long have you been experiencing this?"

"How's your stress level or sleep quality?"

And then, they end up the appointment by prescribing you some medication or a long-term expensive treatment.

The medical industry is a business, patients are customers. The "solution" is often some sort of drug. It's one big legal drug empire.

Walter White's biggest rival.

"Doctors spend only 20 hours studying nutrition in medical school, and then they spend their whole careers treating illnesses caused by poor nutrition."

-    Some quote I saw on Twitter. And it's true.

This isn't to bash doctors or anyone in the medical field, by the way. The point of all this is to make you realize that the people you're taking advice from simply don't care about your health.

For example, have you ever heard,
"It's unhealthy to eat eggs every day"?
So have I. And that is a blatant lie.

Some of the very people in charge of public health look like they belong in a competitive eating contest rather than a position of medical authority.

This isn't about shaming—it's about common sense. If someone can't manage their own health, why should they be making decisions about yours?

If you're trying to break free from cocaine addiction, you're not going to seek advice from the cocaine addict, know what I mean?

Are all doctors evil? Absolutely not.
Do they heal people? At times, often they do not.
The system isn't broken; it's designed that way.

During fasting, your insulin sensitivity is heightened. When you consume sugary or high-carb (processed carbs) foods like cereals, your blood sugar rises rapidly. A **sharp insulin spike**, leads to a rapid drop in blood sugar later (hypoglycemia), making you feel tired, sluggish, and hungry again soon after. Increased cravings for more carbs and sugar throughout the day. Potential for insulin resistance over time if this pattern becomes frequent.

This is why you're always hungry, bloated, and tired. Insulin is a hormone that reduces blood sugar by getting sugar out of the blood and also puts it in the cells.

The more sugar you consume, the more sugar you crave. If you keep eating more sugar, your body will start protecting itself and blocking receptors for insulin so the sugar doesn't get in. Over time, insulin will rise higher, pushing your blood sugar down, and your blood sugar will become lower than normal.

So now, you have low blood sugar and you're developing more **insulin resistance.** What happens is, the protection mechanism breaks down and stops working. Your insulin starts going down because you can't produce insulin anymore.

Insulin exists to lower your blood sugars but if there's no more insulin production, guess what happens now? Your blood sugar gets higher and higher and that's what you call: **Diabetes. Yes, exactly; it is the disease that generates billions annually.** Once you catch it, it's basically a life-long commitment. The diabetes is married to you, and unlike most marriages today, there's no divorce. Until death does you guys apart.

This is why people with type 1 and 2 diabetes inject themselves with insulin. The best way to hook somebody up for that condition is to make them believe that they need to eat junk as soon as they wake up otherwise, they're going to gain weight, be unfocused, lose muscles, be tired, and not prepared for the rest of the day.

IN SUMMARY

What you eat first will set you up for the rest of the day, it's true. But what you eat first doesn't have to be in the morning.

If you start with sugar and refined carbs, your blood sugar will spike, and your body will release a surge of insulin to bring it down. This often results in crashes that leave you hungry and less energized soon after. Remember, the more sugar you consume, the more you will crave.

Breaking your fast with sugar or processed carbs forces the body to switch to glucose metabolism quickly. It halts fat burning and encourages fat storage, especially around the abdominal area.

Often, we mistake hunger for thirst, and if we hydrate well in the morning, we will be **less** hungry.
Sometimes, when we experience hunger pangs, it's not a genuine need for nourishment but rather our body's digestive processes at work.

Allowing the digestive system to rest through practices like fasting can be beneficial. Fasting initiates autophagy, a natural

process where the body cleanses damaged cells and regenerates new ones, promoting cellular health.
This is why not eating in the morning and prolonging your fast is so beneficial.

There's nothing unhealthy about not eating in the morning. If you're not used to it, it may make you tired and hungry, but who cares? You won't die; as far as I and many experts know, it adds years to your life—proven and experienced.

But keep this in mind: if you want the fast to be effective, you must break it correctly. Eating sugar, cereal, and junk food for breakfast (like you see in advertisements) is definitely not adding years to your life; it's robbing you of them.

If you delay your first meal, your body continues to burn stored fat for energy instead of relying on incoming food. Autophagy continues to do its work as the fast goes on.

If you adopt fasting as a long-term practice, your old cells die and are replaced by new cells, which results in fewer cravings, better skin, more human growth hormone production, improved libido, improved testosterone, reduced cortisol, improved mood, maintained bone density, and an improved overall sense of wellness and health in the long run.

If you want to lose weight, intermittent fasting, OMAD, and regular exercise **(including exercise while fasting)** will help you achieve your goal effectively. You won't even need to track calories like a maniac.

Fasting is not just physical; it's mental as well. It takes discipline not to break a fast under temptation.

Here's a variety of fasting approaches

Intermittent Fasting (IF)

Intermittent fasting cycles between periods of eating and fasting. It doesn't restrict what you eat but when you eat.

Common Intermittent Fasting Methods:

16/8 Method:

Fast for 16 hours, eat within an 8-hour window (e.g., only eating from 12 PM to 8 PM).

18/6 Method:

Fast for 18 hours, eat within a 6-hour window.

20/4 (Warrior Diet):

Fast for 20 hours, eat within a 4-hour window.

Often includes one big meal per day.

OMAD (One Meal A Day):

23-hour fast, eating all calories in one single meal.

It can be extreme but maximizes fat burning and autophagy.

Benefits: Boosts fat burning, improves insulin sensitivity, enhances focus, and simplifies eating.

Prolonged (Extended) Fasting

Prolonged fasting involves fasting for more than 24 hours to cleanse the body and promote healing deeply.

24-Hour Fast:

A full-day fast, also called "Dinner-to-Dinner" fasting.

36-Hour Fast:

A deeper reset forcing the body to burn fat stores.

48-Hour Fast:

Boosts autophagy (cell repair) and depletes glycogen stores.

72-Hour Fast (3-Day Fast):

Deep detox and immune system regeneration.

Recommended occasionally for long-term health benefits.

Benefits: Strong autophagy, improved gut health, enhanced metabolic reset, and reduced inflammation.

Alternate-Day Fasting (ADF)

Eat one day, fast the next, repeat.

Some versions allow up to 500 calories on fasting days.

Helps with weight loss, insulin sensitivity, and longevity.

Benefits: Effective for weight loss and balancing hormones while allowing flexibility.

Dry Fasting (No Food, No Water)

Soft Dry Fasting: No food, but some water (often for religious reasons).

Hard Dry Fasting: No food, no water (most intense).

Absolute Dry Fasting: No food, water, or contact with water (e.g., no showers).

Intermittent Dry Fasting: A mix of dry fasting and water fasting.

Benefits: Stronger autophagy than water fasting, reduces inflammation and burns fat quickly.

Warning: Dry fasting is extreme and should be done with caution and not for extended periods.

Water Fasting

Only water, no food.

It can last from 24 hours to several days or even weeks (some people do 40 days).

Triggers deep autophagy and gut healing.

Benefits: Enhances metabolism, boosts growth hormone, and repairs cells.

Fasting Mimicking Diet (FMD)

Very low-calorie diet (about 500-800 calories/day).

Allows some food while keeping the benefits of fasting.

Benefits: Easier to sustain than full fasting while still gaining some autophagy benefits.

Fasting has a direct impact on **sleep patterns and energy levels**. Many people notice that during prolonged fasts, they sleep **less** yet feel **more energized**.

This happens because the body enters a **regeneration state during sleep**, repairing cells and restoring energy. However, when fasting, the body **mimics this same regeneration process**, leading to increased alertness and a reduced need for sleep. Even a short **1–2-hour** nap can feel deeply refreshing due to the body's heightened repair mechanisms.

At the same time, some fasters experience **more sleep rather than less**, especially when dehydrated. **Dry fasting (no food or water)** can lead to **temporary fatigue**, making rest more appealing.

The body conserves energy when water intake is restricted, which is why some people **sleep more during extended fasts**. However, energy levels **return quickly once rehydrated and often increase beyond normal levels**.

A common concern about fasting is **muscle loss**. The truth is the body prioritizes burning **fat for energy** and only starts breaking down muscle in **prolonged fasts (5+ days of water fasting or extreme calorie restriction)**. Short-term fasting, including intermittent, 24-hour, and even **48-hour fasts**, **preserves muscle while accelerating fat loss** by releasing **growth hormone** and improving insulin sensitivity.

Long-term fasting (5+ days) can eventually lower testosterone **(rises back when done)**, but short-term fasting (12-48 hours) is actually beneficial for testosterone production.

Fasting temporarily raises testosterone and cortisol, helping your body stay alert and burn fat. When you break the fast, these levels naturally drop, but they don't have to go lower than before—it all depends on how you refeed.

If you fuel up with whole foods, healthy fats, and protein, testosterone can actually stabilize at a higher level. However, if you break your fast with junk, refined carbs, and sugar, your hormones will crash, making you feel worse.

Cortisol spikes during fasting to keep you energized, but it normalizes after eating—this is why proper refeeding is key to maintaining optimal hormone balance. Nutrients, Not Junk

Dry fasting (no food or water) should be approached with caution. While a 1-day dry fast is often easier and more beneficial than a 2-day water fast, going beyond 48 hours without water is not recommended unless one has prior experience.

Dry fasting causes the body to enter a **deep detox state**, eliminating damaged cells faster than water fasting.

However, if done irresponsibly, dehydration can become a serious risk. Beginners should start with shorter dry fasts and gradually and carefully increase their duration.

Fasting Tips for Beginners

Stay Hydrated – But Don't Overdo It

During water fasting, drink when you feel thirsty or hungry—not just for the sake of drinking.

Too much water can flush out essential minerals, leading to dizziness, fatigue, or electrolyte imbalances.

Balance Electrolytes – Use Salt & Lemon Water Wisely

Adding a pinch of Himalayan salt to water helps prevent sodium depletion and headaches.

Lemon water is great for detox support and taste variation but avoid excessive lemon as it can stimulate digestion and make fasting harder.

Rotate between plain water and lemon water to keep hydration balanced.

Hunger Comes in Waves – Ride Them Out

Drinking warm water, herbal tea, or salt water can help suppress cravings.

If you feel extreme hunger, distract yourself with activities like walking, reading, or deep breathing.

Don't Fear Fatigue – Energy Will Come

Feeling a little weak or sluggish during the first 24-48 hours is normal.

After this, your body switches to fat-burning mode, and energy levels increase naturally.

Rest, But Stay Active

Light movement like walking, stretching, or yoga helps circulate energy and reduce fatigue.

Avoid intense workouts during extended fasts (3+ days), as your body is in recovery mode.

Sleep Adjustments – Expect Changes

Some people need less sleep while fasting because their bodies are in a self-repair mode, similar to deep sleep. Others, especially if dehydrated, may sleep more. Listen to your body.

Dry Fasting – Shorter is Stronger, Less is More

A 24-hour dry fast is often easier and more beneficial than a 48-hour water fast.

More than 48 hours of dry fasting should only be attempted with experience and knowledge.

Break dry fasts gently. To avoid shocking the system, start with sips of water, followed by fruit or broth.

Break Your Fast Correctly – No Junk Food!

The first foods after fasting should be easy to digest:

Best choices: Fruits, bone broth, lightly cooked vegetables, eggs.

Worst choices: Processed food, greasy meals, and high-sugar foods.

Expect Detox Symptoms – But Don't Panic

Headaches, fatigue, dizziness, or nausea can happen as toxins leave the body.

Drink salt water, herbal teas, or lemon water to ease symptoms.

Food is a nourishment to the body. If it doesn't do any good to your body, it's not food; it's junk.

Fasting Is a Tool – Use It Wisely

Fasting is not about starving but about healing, discipline, and resetting your system.

For example, if you feel like you've been eating a lot of junk lately, fasting is the best way to detox.

It's not a competition—listen to your body, and stop if you feel unwell.

The more you practice fasting, the easier it gets and the better you feel.

Also, try not to beat yourself up too much if you break your fast under the temptation of hunger.
It happens to the best of us.

Eye-Opening.

As you research and open your mind to the truth, you'll realize that much of what we've been taught is built on deception— lies designed to control, not to help us thrive.

These falsehoods don't exist by accident. They are crafted, promoted, and reinforced by industries that profit from your ignorance and poor health. Wickedness and greed drive the system, not your well-being.

Think about it—if they can control how you eat, how you think, and how you live, they can ensure that you remain sick, dependent, and profitable. A sick person isn't just someone struggling with their health; they are a customer—a lifelong patient trapped in a cycle of medication, medical visits, and false solutions.

Take fasting, for example.
We've been led to believe that fasting is dangerous, unnecessary, or even harmful. But if you look beyond the surface and take even a moment to research, you'll find that the opposite is true. Fasting heals. It allows the body to reset, repair, and cleanse itself in ways that no drug ever could.

And yet, there's plenty of rumors about it being potentially unhealthy—why? Because a person who fasts regularly is not a profitable patient. They can't charge you for it. *Remember, if it doesn't make money, it doesn't make sense.*

And what about the infamous "three meals a day" rule? You've been told that eating three meals a day—plus snacks—is the key to good health. But let's be honest—most people don't eat because they are truly hungry.

They eat out of gluttony, addiction, and habit. They eat because food tastes good, comforts them, and is available—not because their body actually needs it. Gluttony is a major killer. It fuels obesity, diabetes, heart disease, and countless other conditions that keep the medical industry thriving.

As I told you earlier in this book,
I ate after that fast, not because I was hungry, but because the food tasted good. I was well-hydrated; my body had what it needed, but I still wanted more. And what happened? I vomited. My body rejected what my mind desired. Train your mind, and your body will be thankful.

That moment was a lesson—a painful but necessary reminder that mindset is everything. Your cravings, your habits, your so-called "hunger"—most of it is mental, not physical. If you don't control your mind, it will control you.

The Truth About Nutrition and Lifestyle: A Profitable Lie
If you still believe that eating first thing in the morning is necessary for health, understand this: that idea was not created by science.

It was created by marketing. It was pushed by food companies, cereal manufacturers, industries that profit when you blindly consume, and even schools. And most people? They don't even question it. They eat because they've been conditioned to, and in doing so, they are slowly harming themselves. Just as planned.

The hard truth is that the modern food and medical industries were never designed to keep you healthy. They were built to keep you sick enough to need them, but alive enough to keep buying their solutions. They don't want you to be independent. They don't want you thinking for yourself. They want you obedient, dependent, and willing to believe whatever they tell you.

But now that you know the truth, what will you do with it? Will you continue to eat the way they programmed you to? Will you keep believing their lies? Or will you take control of your health, your body, and your mind—before it's too late?

The choice is yours.

My favorite part of the

"I Was An MIT Educated Neurosurgeon Now I'm Unemployed And Alone In The Mountains How Did I Get There?"

YouTube video from the **_Goobie and Doobie_** channel (this is the last time I mention this video, I promise) was when he made the leaky roof analogy. It explains perfectly how the system operates.

Analogy (from Goobie)

Let's say your house has a leaky roof that is causing water damage. You can clearly see the damage. The repair workers might replace the drywall, remove the insulation, install new insulation, and paint the walls a nice color. However, they are not addressing the underlying issue—the leaky roof itself.

What do you think will happen? Eventually, the homeowners will need to call the workers again because new water damage will occur. Why? Because they didn't address the root cause of the problem; instead, they only performed a temporary fix.

Explanation (from me)

Over time, the homeowner continues to call the repair workers. Each time, the men come to repair the house without fixing the source of the problem (the leak). They only set up a temporary fix until the problem resurfaces so they can return as the only solution and get paid again. As a result, the house's condition worsens with each repair until it reaches a point where it can no longer be fixed.

Don't take advice from the repair workers who patiently wait for your call so they can make more money without ever putting you out of your misery for good.

They don't care about the state of your house; they just want your money. If they address the source of your problems, you won't be useful to them because you won't be a customer anymore.

For the slow-headed, this isn't about houses.

A patient cured is a lost customer.

The breakfast hoax is one of the biggest lies ever sold to you. But now that you know the truth, you can take back control. Choose nutrient-dense foods, start fasting, listen to your body, and stop following the food industry's agenda.

Your health is your responsibility. No more blindly trusting corporations or falling for marketing traps! Marketing plays on people's emotions, habits, and comfort to keep them hooked on junk food.

They want you addicted. They want you weak. They want you to seek comfort in processed foods when you're stressed, sad, or tired. But you have the power to break the cycle. Food should nourish, not control you.

There is so much promotion of junk food and all sorts of drinks, sugar, and seed oils. All these destructive atrocities are basically unavoidable. And then, you look at the amount of money they make by treating people and you see clearly.

It's not a coincidence. It's a billion-dollar business, one that involves partnerships and publicity.

Your health is worth more than anything; take care of it. Don't entrust it to those who profit from your sickness.

Enlightenment

Cultures, Religions, and Traditions.

Hara Hachi Bu: The Okinawan Secret to Longevity

Okinawa, Japan, is one of the world's **Blue Zones**—regions where people live significantly longer and healthier lives. One of their key lifestyle habits is **Hara Hachi Bu**, a mindful eating practice that translates to **"eat until you are 80% full."**

Instead of eating until they feel stuffed, Okinawans stop when they are satisfied but not completely full, giving their digestive system room to process food without strain.

This method naturally reduces **caloric intake**, which has been linked to increased longevity and a lower risk of diseases like **obesity, diabetes, and heart disease**.

Research suggests that **eating fewer calories while maintaining high nutritional quality** can slow aging and reduce inflammation. Unlike restrictive diets, **Hara Hachi Bu is not about deprivation but about balance**—listening to the body's natural hunger signals and stopping before overeating.

If someone told me I could only use 3 words to describe what America isn't, I would go: *"Hara Hachi Bu."*

Buddhist Mindful Eating (Various Countries) – Eating with Awareness & Gratitude

Buddhist monks practice **silent eating (Oryoki in Japan and Thudong in Thailand)** to fully experience the food's **flavors, textures, and purpose**.

Meals are seen as **a sacred gift, not an indulgence**—consumed slowly and with full attention.

Many monks practice **eating one meal a day before noon**, allowing the body to rest and fast naturally. Overeating is seen as **feeding desires rather than nourishing the body**.

You notice something after a prolonged fast. Fasting reveals a truth that modern society often ignores—**food is a blessing, not an indulgence.**

When you fast, you gain a new perspective on hunger and appreciation. In a world where food is always available, we become picky, entitled, and ungrateful, treating meals as comfort, entertainment, or habit rather than the life-sustaining nourishment they are.

But when you fast, something shifts. Suddenly, the foods you once ignored or disliked become appealing. If you're dry fasting and thirst begins to take over, even something as simple as a cucumber becomes a gift rather than a burden.

And when you finally break your fast, you truly taste your food again. The textures, flavors, and aromas become more intense and satisfying, reminding you that eating is meant to nourish, not numb.

Most of you reading this don't eat because you're hungry—you eat because you're bored. How often have you reached for junk food just because you're watching a movie? How often do you eat simply because it's "time to eat" rather than because your body actually needs fuel?

The truth is most people have a food addiction, but they don't recognize it. If you can't go 24 hours drinking only water, you might want to ask yourself—who's in control? You or your cravings?

Breaking Free from the Gluttony Trap

Fasting is **not as difficult as people make it seem**. Here's a simple way to complete a **24-hour water fast** with ease:

Eat at noon.
Drink only water for the rest of the day.
Sleep for 8 hours—one-third of the fast is already done.
Wake up at 6, 7, or 8 AM. You have only 4–6 hours left before breaking your fast.

With **a little drive and discipline, it's absolutely achievable**—and once you complete it, you'll realize how much power you actually have over your body.

Modern society encourages gluttony, but self-control is the real thing. When you master fasting, you master yourself. People are making an entertainment out of eating junk. It's wild.

Discipline Over **Gluttony**. Purpose Over **Pleasure**.

Ayurvedic Eating: Food as Medicine (India)

Ayurveda, an **ancient Indian holistic health system**, treats **food as medicine** and emphasizes **balance, digestion, and eating according to body type (Doshas).**

Key Principles

Eat **whole, fresh, natural foods** instead of processed junk.

Chew thoroughly and eat slowly to aid digestion.

Avoid overeating—overeating is believed to create "Ama" (toxins) in the body.

Eat with awareness and gratitude, seeing food as nourishment rather than indulgence.

This system focuses on **how food affects the body long-term rather than just its taste.**

The Mediterranean Diet: Eating Like the Ancients (Greece, Italy, Spain)

The Mediterranean diet is considered one of the healthiest in the world, reducing the risk of heart disease, obesity, and diabetes.

Key Practices

Meals are social and slow-paced, preventing mindless eating.

Olive oil, vegetables, fish, and whole grains dominate the diet instead of processed foods.

Smaller portions are naturally satisfying, avoiding overconsumption.

Eating in a relaxed, social environment enhances digestion, mood, and long-term health.

Confucian Eating Philosophy: Balance & Harmony (China)

Confucianism teaches that **everything, including food, must be balanced.**

Key Principles

Eat in moderation and avoid excess.

Meals should be varied but balanced (proteins, vegetables, grains).

Chopsticks encourage smaller bites and **slower eating,** which prevents overeating. **Avoid heavy foods at night** to aid digestion.

Hadza Tribe Eating: Eating Only When Needed (Tanzania)

The **African Hadza tribe** still follows a **hunter-gatherer lifestyle,** similar to **early humans.**

Key Practices

No fixed meal schedule—they eat **only when hungry**, not out of habit.

No processed foods—only fresh, natural foods.

Fasting happens naturally when food is scarce, keeping metabolism efficient.

This natural approach **prevents obesity, diabetes, and metabolic disorders** seen in modern societies.

The Korean "Bansang" Tradition: Balanced & Intentional Eating (South Korea)

Bansang refers to **a traditional Korean meal setup**, where **many small side dishes (banchan)** accompany rice and soup.

Why This Prevents Overeating:

Diverse dishes prevent cravings and promote satiety with smaller portions.

Meals are balanced with proteins, vegetables, and fermented foods, supporting gut health.

Slow eating with chopsticks and soups naturally limits overconsumption.

By structuring meals this way, **overeating becomes unlikely.**

Modern Society Ignores These Principles

Today's Western diet promotes constant eating, oversized portions, and processed food.

Ancient traditions focused on moderation, balance, and self-control—leading to healthier, longer lives.

What is the result of abandoning these principles? Modern societies face obesity, diabetes, and chronic diseases.

Eat mindfully, stop before you're full, and choose real food over processed junk.

Stop the junk or the junk will stop you. (your heart)

The Silent Epidemic: Gluttony, Poisoned Food, and the Decline of Health

Gluttony has become a silent, insidious killer, one that feeds on the ignorance of an entire society. For the first time in history, children today may potentially have a lower life expectancy than their parents—and it's not because of a disease or natural disaster but because we have created a system where toxic food is the norm.

This isn't just about overconsumption—it's about the deliberate poisoning of our youth. Sugar, artificial colorings like Red 40, toxic seed oils, and chemical dyes are all hidden in plain sight, filling the shelves of our supermarkets and destroying the health of our children. These are not just "empty calories"— they are silent killers, silently eroding their bodies from the inside.

The impact is staggering. Infertility rates are rising, and our children are being fed chemicals that disrupt their hormonal balance, making them more vulnerable to chronic illnesses, mental health issues, and early deaths. This generation's obesity rates are skyrocketing while the quality of their food is plummeting.

The food that's meant to nourish us has become nothing more than a weapon of mass destruction. What we once called "food" now barely resembles anything the body can use—it's simply poison in disguise.

We've normalized feeding our kids processed, sugary snacks while their bodies slowly deteriorate. They're eating products with addictive sugar that cause hyperactivity and make them more susceptible to mental health disorders.

And then the cycle begins. These children, instead of being taught how to nourish themselves properly, are labeled with ADHD—a condition caused by the very food they're fed.

They're prescribed drugs that numb their natural happiness and energy, all while the pharmaceutical industry profits off their illness. The medical industry feeds off the very problems it creates.

The solution is never prevention; it's simply more medication, treatment, and profits. The food industry creates the problem, and the medical industry offers the "cure," but the truth is that the cure isn't a pill; it's in the choices we make daily about what we eat. We are being sold poison, and the ones who profit from it are making a killing, literally, at the expense of our health.

If we don't take control now, we are handing future generations a broken system where they are born into a world where obesity, infertility, and mental health crises are the norm.

It's time to wake up and stop being complicit in our own destruction. The food we consume should nourish, heal, and energize us, but we've let it become a tool of control and profit for industries that don't care about our well-being. We've been deceived, and it's time to demand the truth.

Knowing what to eat is not rocket science,

If it doesn't nourish your body, it isn't food.

A True Relationship with Food

In the regions where people live the longest and healthiest lives, food is not treated as entertainment, comfort, or addiction. Instead, it is seen for what it truly is: fuel, nourishment, and a tool for longevity.

Unlike modern societies, where eating is driven by cravings, emotional dependence, and convenience, Blue Zone cultures have deep-rooted traditions that promote mindful eating, balance, and self-control.

These communities—from the Okinawans in Japan to the Ikarians in Greece—prioritize whole, unprocessed foods and consume them in moderation. Their diets are rich in nutrients, not chemicals, and they follow principles like Hara Hachi Bu (eating until 80% full) to avoid overindulgence.

Unlike Western cultures that binge on processed foods, Blue Zones understand that food isn't food if it doesn't nourish the body.

Beyond nutrition, these cultures also prioritize movement, social connections, and stress management, all of which contribute to their overall health and longevity. They don't just eat well—they live well.

On the other hand, the modern world has corrupted the purpose of food. It is marketed as a source of pleasure rather than survival, leading to a society plagued by obesity, metabolic disorders, and chronic diseases. Blue Zones serve as a reminder of what we've lost—that food should heal, not harm.

It's not just about what you eat—it's about how you view food. If you see it as fuel, it will serve you. If you see it as comfort, it will control you.

If people truly understood how to eat, what to eat, and how often to eat, we would eliminate at least 70% of modern health problems;

diabetes, chronic inflammation, acne, fatigue, cancer, Alzheimer's, bloating, insulin resistance, sleep disorders, gut issues, vitamin deficiencies, hair loss, infertility, low testosterone, brain fog, and even heart disease. Nearly every major illness can be traced back to **poor nutrition, overconsumption, and toxic food choices.**

If the average person knew how to use food as fuel instead of comfort, they wouldn't be trapped in a cycle of lifelong medications, surgeries, and constant health struggles.

What you eat determines your energy, focus, hormones, skin, fertility, mental clarity, and longevity. The modern diet isn't just unhealthy—it's a carefully crafted system to keep you weak, overweight, and in need of "treatments."

Breakfasting

Nutrients, Not Junk.

As we talked about earlier,

Your body is a temple that requires attention and care. It needs to be nourished with healthy nutrients, not junk. Remember that each time you eat in the morning, you are breaking a fast.

Both fasting and breaking the fast are equally important. Society has conditioned you to begin your day with unhealthy choices, often loaded with sugar and processed foods. It's one big club, if they push you to eat unhealthily, you become unhealthy, and since you're smart, you already know who profits from the unhealthy.

Eating processed carbs, sugar, and junk food first thing in the morning is one of the worst things you can do for your body. While it may seem harmless, it gradually undermines your metabolism, energy levels, hormones, and overall health.

Here's what happens in the long run:

Blood Sugar Spikes & Crashes—Eating sugary cereals, pastries, and carb-heavy breakfasts spikes insulin, giving you a short burst of energy.

This is followed by a hard crash, leaving you tired, sluggish, and craving more sugar. This cycle leads to insulin resistance, which is the gateway to diabetes, weight gain, and metabolic dysfunction.

Chronic Inflammation & Disease – Processed breakfast foods loaded with seed oils, refined sugars, and preservatives trigger chronic inflammation, a root cause of heart disease, cancer, joint pain, autoimmune disorders, and neurological decline (like Alzheimer's).

Hormonal Imbalances & Testosterone Decline—Starting your day with sugar and processed carbs elevates cortisol (the stress hormone) and lowers testosterone over time. This results in fat gain, mood swings, low energy, and weak muscle growth.

Gut Damage & Poor Digestion – Constantly eating refined grains, sugars, and processed foods weakens your gut lining, leading to bloating, indigestion, IBS, leaky gut, and poor nutrient absorption. Over time, this can cause food intolerances, vitamin deficiencies, and even brain fog.

Increased Risk of Obesity & Fat Storage – Your body is most insulin-sensitive in the morning, meaning any junk food you eat is quickly stored as fat instead of being used for energy. Over time, this leads to stubborn belly fat, obesity, and a slowed metabolism.

Higher Risk of Heart Disease & Diabetes – Consuming sugar-packed breakfast foods daily raises triglycerides, cholesterol, and blood pressure. This directly contributes to heart disease, strokes, and type 2 diabetes—all preventable if you just stop eating garbage in the morning, or at all.

Your body is in a highly sensitive state, ready to absorb nutrients efficiently—this is your opportunity to refuel with the best possible foods to promote healing, energy, and longevity.

If you've only fasted overnight, your body doesn't need a slow reintroduction—you can go straight into eating. However, it's still best to start with hydration first, followed by whole, nutrient-dense foods.

One-Day Dry Fast (24 Hours) – Hydration First, Then Light Foods

After 24 hours without food and water, your body is dehydrated and needs careful rehydration.
Start with water. Take small sips, and don't chug. (add lemon to replenish electrolytes)

Fresh fruit (water-rich ones like watermelon, oranges, grapes, cucumbers, or papaya) provides hydration, fiber, and natural sugars to wake up digestion gently.

Bone broth. Loaded with minerals and gentle on the stomach.

After 30–60 minutes of hydration, you can eat a small, easily digestible meal—such as steamed vegetables, soft-boiled eggs, or a light protein source like fish or chicken.

Avoid Heavy, greasy meals, dairy, or processed foods—they stress digestion.

Two-Day Dry Fast (48 Hours). SLOW Hydration, Then Gradual Eating

After two days of no food or water, your body is in deep repair mode and needs a careful approach to refeeding.

Start with a glass of water, taken in small sips over 10–15 minutes.

After thirty minutes to an hour, introduce hydrating fruits (watermelon, papaya, or oranges).

After another 30–60 minutes, eat soft, fiber-rich foods like steamed veggies, smoothies, or bone broth.

Protein should be added last—eggs, fish, or lean chicken in small portions.

Warning: Eating too much too quickly after a long, dry fast can cause digestive distress, vomiting, bloating, or, in extreme cases, refeeding syndrome. (Like the woman who ate 23 bananas after fasting for 7 days.)

Why Hydration Comes First

Hydrating properly before eating is crucial, no matter how long you've fasted. When you fast, your body prioritizes cellular repair, and digestion is on "pause."

However, drinking too much water right before eating dilutes stomach acid, making digestion less efficient and leading to bloating and discomfort.

This is why allowing at least 20–30 minutes between hydration and your first meal is important to ensure optimal digestion.

Never Break a Fast with:
Refined Carbs & Sugars – This leads to rapid insulin spikes and crashes.

Fast Food and Processed Junk: After a fast, your body absorbs everything faster, including toxins, chemicals, and inflammatory seed oils.
Heavy, Greasy Meals. Overloads your digestive system and causes discomfort.

The Best Time to Refuel Your Body for Maximum Health

After fasting, this is the time to give it **nutrients—not junk.** Instead of wasting this opportunity on processed carbs and sugars, use it to rebuild strength, optimize energy, and enhance longevity.

Think of your first meal after fasting as your body's "reset button." If you fuel it right, you set yourself up for better digestion, stronger metabolism, and overall better health.

If you fuel it wrong, you undo most of the benefits of fasting and flood your body with unnecessary toxins.

Eat with purpose. Break your fast like your health depends on it—because it does.

The Best Foods to Eat for Breakfast: Fueling Your Morning the Right Way

Breakfast should be about **fueling your body for energy, focus, and longevity**, not just satisfying cravings. The best morning foods are **nutrient-dense, blood sugar-stabilizing, and rich in essential vitamins and minerals** to set you up for a productive day.

Here is a list of powerful, science-backed foods that make for an **optimal breakfast**, whether you are breaking a fast or just starting your morning the right way.

Steak & Red Meat: The Ultimate Protein Source

Myth: Red meat is bad for your health.
Truth: High-quality red meat is one of the most nutrient-dense foods you can eat. It provides essential amino acids, healthy fats, and vital nutrients that support strength, endurance, and cognitive function.

The myth that red meat causes heart disease has been widely debunked—processed foods and sugar are the real culprits behind cardiovascular problems. Red meat contains zinc, which helps the body produce testosterone and is important for the immune system. Contains Iron, which helps in,

Blood cell production: Iron is needed to make new red blood cells and prevent iron deficiency anemia

(blood disorder that occurs when the body lacks healthy red blood cells or hemoglobin to carry oxygen). This is why women need more Iron; they lose blood during menstruation, which can lead to lower iron levels.

Since iron is a key component of hemoglobin (the protein in red blood cells that carries oxygen), losing too much iron can cause fatigue, weakness, and dizziness.

Iron is also essential during pregnancy, as a woman's blood volume increases significantly to supply oxygen to the growing baby. Iron helps transport oxygen throughout the body, improving energy levels, brain function, and focus. For this reason, iron deficiency is often linked to fatigue.

Hormone production: Iron is needed to make some hormones.

Energy production: Iron is a component of enzymes that increase the rate of chemical reactions, including those involved in energy production.

Healthy cells, skin, hair, and nails: Iron helps maintain the health of these tissues.

Muscle function: Iron is a component of myoglobin, a protein that stores oxygen in muscle cells and gives muscles their red color.

Cognitive function: Iron contributes to cognitive function.

Of course, everything in moderation, even good things.

Why it's great:

High in creatine, which enhances brain function and athletic performance.

Rich in heme iron, which is better absorbed than plant-based iron and prevents fatigue.

Contains carnosine, an antioxidant that reduces inflammation and supports metabolism.

Best way to eat it:

Grass-fed steak, ground beef patties, or beef liver for an extra nutrient boost.

Eggs: The Perfect Nutrient Bomb

Myth: Eggs raise cholesterol and increase heart disease risk.

Truth: Eggs contain cholesterol, but it is dietary cholesterol, which does not negatively impact blood cholesterol levels.

In fact, eggs **increase good cholesterol (HDL)** and provide essential nutrients that support heart and brain health.

The brain contains a significant portion of the body's total cholesterol, most of it located in the myelin sheath, the part of the brain primarily made with cholesterol.

This is why eating eggs every day isn't harmful, by the way.

Eggs provide all of the nine essential amino acids (also known as the building blocks of protein), making them an effective food for maintaining, building, and repairing muscle. Why are eggs good for building muscle?

Protein
Eggs contain high-quality protein, which is the building block for muscle.

Leucine
Eggs contain a lot of leucine, an amino acid that helps the body synthesize protein for muscle gain.

Vitamin D
Eggs contain vitamin D, which is important for bone health and may help reduce the risk of muscle impairment.

Energy
The combination of protein and healthy fats in eggs provides a steady release of energy, which can help prevent fatigue during workouts.

Eggs are a good post-workout snack because they help repair and rebuild muscle. Eating eggs before a workout can help your body initiate the muscle-building process.

High-density lipoprotein (HDL), also known as "good" cholesterol, is beneficial because it helps remove other types of cholesterol from the body.

Cholesterol helps produce hormones like estrogen, testosterone, and adrenal hormones, chemicals produced by the adrenal glands that regulate many bodily functions, for example, cortisol or androgens

Adrenal hormones help control:

Blood pressure: Adrenaline and noradrenaline increase blood pressure in response to stress

Blood sugar: Adrenaline and noradrenaline increase blood sugar levels

Metabolism: Adrenal hormones help the body convert food into energy

Stress response: Adrenaline and noradrenaline are part of the body's "fight-or-flight" response

Vitamin D: Cholesterol is essential for the body to produce vitamin D from sunlight

Digestion: Cholesterol helps produce bile acids, which help the body digest fat and absorb nutrients. High HDL cholesterol levels I are linked to a lower risk of heart disease and stroke.

Now you see why they label it **"dangerous-to-eat-daily,"** eggs contain almost every nutrient the body needs. A healthy person isn't profitable, know what I mean

Why it's great:

High in choline, an essential nutrient for brain function and memory.

Contains lutein and zeaxanthin, antioxidants that support eye health.

Loaded with bioavailable protein, perfect for muscle maintenance and repair.

Best way to eat it:

Soft-boiled, scrambled, or as an omelet with vegetables.

Avocados: A Nutrient Powerhouse

Myth: Avocados are high in fat, so they should be avoided. **Truth:** The fats in avocados are monounsaturated, which improve heart health, reduce inflammation, and support brain function. Fat is essential for hormone production and does not make you fat—processed carbs and sugars do.

Why it's great:

Balances blood sugar and keeps energy stable throughout the day.

High in fiber, supporting digestion and gut health.

A great source of potassium is essential for muscle and nerve function.

Heart health. High potassium can help lower blood pressure and reduce the risk of heart disease.

Digestion. They're rich in fiber, which can help with digestion, prevent constipation, help move waste through your body, and keep your bowel movements regular.

Skin health. Avocados contain omega-3 fats and antioxidants that can help reduce inflammation and promote healthy skin.

Eye Health. The superfood contains antioxidants that can help reduce the risk of age-related macular degeneration and cataracts.

Brain Health. They contain folate, which can help produce dopamine, serotonin, and norepinephrine, which regulate mood.

Blood sugar. The fruits contain magnesium, which can help regulate blood sugar levels.

Inflammation. Niacin can help fight inflammation in the body.

Cholesterol. Avocados contain niacin, which can help improve cholesterol and triglyceride levels.

Best way to eat it:

Sliced on eggs, mashed with lime and salt, or blended in a smoothie.

Berries: The Antioxidant Powerhouses

Myth: Fruit has too much sugar and should be avoided.
Truth: The natural sugars in fruit are accompanied by fiber, antioxidants, and vitamins that prevent the insulin spikes caused by processed sugar. Berries, in particular, are packed with nutrients.

Why they're great:

Antioxidants protect us against oxidative stress, slowing aging and reducing disease risk by neutralizing free radicals, which are unstable molecules that damage cells and contribute to aging.

Compounds in wild blueberry leaves may help reduce inflammation that plays a role in cognitive brain disorders like Alzheimer's disease, supporting brain health and cognitive function.

We just talked about the role of Iron. Well, some berries can inhibit iron absorption. However, you can pair iron-rich foods with foods high in vitamin C to help your body absorb more iron.

Some berries are high in vitamin C, strawberries, blueberries, raspberries, and blackberries.

They also help regulate blood sugar, making them a great source of carbohydrates. There are healthy carbs and processed carbs.

"Healthy carbs" refer to unprocessed, whole grains and fiber-rich carbohydrates found in foods like fruits, vegetables, legumes, and whole grains.

In contrast, "processed carbs" are refined carbohydrates that have been stripped of their fiber and nutrients through processing, like white bread, white rice, and sugary drinks.

These carbs lead to a quicker blood sugar spike and less nutritional value, which, over time, unavoidably leads to diseases.

Fiber slows down the absorption of sugar into the bloodstream by slowing down digestion, which helps prevent blood sugar spikes. Soluble fiber, in particular, dissolves in water and forms a gel-like substance in the stomach, further hindering the rapid absorption of sugar.

This is why fruits, although they contain sugar, contain high amounts of fiber, vitamins, and antioxidants. These make them healthy and energizing instead of making you sluggish, bloated, and fatigued like processed carbs that give you insulin spikes.

Best way to eat them:

Mixed with Greek yogurt, in a smoothie, or on their own with nuts. Simple is best; you can also eat them on their own.

Greek Yogurt & Kefir: Gut-Healing Probiotics

Myth: All dairy is bad for you.
Truth: Low-quality, processed dairy can cause inflammation,

but fermented dairy like Greek yogurt and kefir is rich in probiotics, healthy fats, and protein, which support gut health and digestion.

Why it's great:

Boosts gut microbiome, improving digestion and immune function.

The Gut Microbiome is useful for;

Digestion. The gut microbiome produces enzymes that break down carbohydrates and other nutrients

Immune system. The gut microbiome helps train the immune system

Protection. The gut microbiome protects against harmful bacteria and pathogens

Vitamin production. The gut microbiome produces vitamins like biotin and vitamin K

Hormone production. The gut microbiome produces hormones that help the body store fat

The food you eat introduces new microbes to your gut microbiome. A healthy gut microbiome can reduce the risk of obesity, heart disease, diabetes, and cancer.

Rich in protein and calcium, it is essential for bone and muscle health.

Contains CLA (conjugated linoleic acid), which supports fat metabolism.

Best way to eat it:

Plain, unsweetened Greek yogurt with berries, with honey, natural plant powder supplements, or mixed with cinnamon.

Nuts & Seeds: Nutrient-Dense Energy Boosters

Myth: Nuts are too high in fat and calories.
Truth: Nuts contain healthy fats that stabilize blood sugar, support brain function, and reduce inflammation. They are also rich in fiber, vitamins, and essential minerals.

Why they're great:

Almonds and walnuts support brain health and reduce inflammation.

Walnuts: Contain nutrients like vitamin E, selenium, and zinc that can help prevent skin aging, which is why cold-press virgin olive oil is so good for the skin, the scalp, and the body in general; it is rich in vitamin E.

Vitamin E is a fat-soluble vitamin that acts as an antioxidant and helps the body produce red blood cells. It's found in many foods, oils, and fats. How vitamin E is important:

Cell regeneration. Vitamin E helps cells regenerate and supports the immune system

Antioxidant. Vitamin E neutralizes free radicals that can damage cells and contribute to cancer and cardiovascular disease

Anti-inflammatory. Vitamin E can reduce inflammation and make skin look younger

Nerve regeneration. Vitamin E deficiency can lead to degenerative changes in the nervous system and decreased nerve regeneration

Cell membrane repair. Vitamin E is important for repairing cell membranes, including myocyte cell membranes

Best way to eat them:

A handful of mixed nuts, blended in smoothies or sprinkled on yogurt.

Wild-Caught Salmon & Fatty Fish: Omega-3 Brain Fuel

Myth: Fish is not an ideal breakfast food.
Truth: For centuries, cultures worldwide have included fish in breakfast. Fatty fish provides high-quality protein and omega-3s, which reduce inflammation and improve brain function.

Why it's great:

Reduces inflammation and supports joint health.

Boosts cognitive function and mental clarity.

Improves mood and energy levels.

Fish is a good source of protein and omega-3 fatty acids, which can help lower blood pressure and reduce the risk of heart disease.

Fish is rich in calcium and phosphorus and a great source of minerals, such as iron, zinc, iodine, magnesium, and potassium.

Best way to eat it:

Smoked salmon with eggs, eaten with rice, grilled salmon with avocado, or mixed into an omelet.

Bone Broth: Liquid Gold for Healing

Myth: Bone broth is just another health trend.

Truth: Bone broth has been used for centuries in traditional cultures as a healing elixir. It is packed with minerals, collagen, and amino acids that support overall health.

Why it's great:

Rich in collagen and gelatin, which repair joints, skin, and gut lining.

Collagen is the most abundant protein in the human body, making up about 30% of total protein content.

It plays a structural role in skin, bones, joints, muscles, and connective tissues, keeping the body strong, flexible, and resilient.

Intermittent fasting (IF) can increase collagen production, which can help improve skin elasticity and firmness.

As we age, collagen production naturally declines, leading to wrinkles, joint pain, weaker bones, and slower recovery. This is why maintaining collagen can provide powerful health longevity.

As collagen levels drop with age, the skin loses firmness, sags, and becomes more prone to wrinkles. This is why many anti-aging supplements and skincare products focus on increasing collagen production.

Collagen is often recommended for athletes, older adults, and people recovering from injuries to promote joint flexibility and faster healing. It can help those experiencing hair loss, slow hair growth, or brittle nails due to aging or nutrient deficiencies.

It helps repair the intestinal lining, which is crucial for gut health. It may **also reduce symptoms of leaky gut syndrome**, IBS, and inflammation. It supports digestion by promoting **stomach acid production and gut microbiome balance**.

Collagen's role in gut health is especially important for people with **autoimmune diseases, food sensitivities, or chronic digestive issues**.

It helps **support lean muscle growth and faster recovery**, making it a valuable addition to an **athlete's nutrition plan**.

Collagen deficiency can contribute to **weakened arteries**, increasing the risk of cardiovascular diseases, which is a key reason why older people tend to experience more cardiovascular issues.

Bone broth contains essential amino acids that aid in digestion.

Boosts hydration and replaces lost electrolytes.

Best way to eat it:

Sipped warm in the morning or used in soups and stews.

Foods to Avoid in the Morning (Almost everything they claim as a healthy breakfast)

Refined Carbs (Cereals, White Bread, Bagels, Pastries) – Cause insulin spikes, leading to energy crashes and fat storage.

Sugary Yogurts & Smoothies – Most contain more sugar than soda, wrecking metabolism.

Processed Meats (Bacon, Sausage with Additives) – Full of preservatives and harmful nitrates.

Seed Oils (Canola, Soy, Vegetable Oil) – Cause inflammation and long-term health issues.

Breakfast Bars & Packaged "Health Foods" are often loaded with sugar, artificial ingredients, and low-quality protein.

Most people consume all five for breakfast on a daily basis and wonder why they feel like a deflated balloon as early as 60. But 60 isn't old; you can live up to 120. In theory.

People get sick in their later years because their bad choices, lack of discipline, and neglect are catching up to them.

You're not sick because you're old; you're old because you're sick, and you're sick because of the poison you eat on a daily basis for years, adding up to decades, robbing you decades of your existence.

If people had educated themselves, most health complications and diseases would have gone away. Blindly taking advice from an evil billion-dollar industry is not education; reading this book and doing your research is; congrats to you.

A two-liter bottle of orange soda can contain up to 55 grams of sugar per 1 ½ cup (375 milliliters). The average cup holds 240 milliliters, meaning that if you drink just three cups in one evening, you've consumed over 100 grams of sugar in a few hours—without even noticing.

But that's not all. Add in breakfast cereals, cookies, bread, fruit juice, and processed snacks, and your sugar intake skyrockets to over 200 grams in one day. Compare that to the recommended daily limit:

36 grams for men
25 grams for women

The average person consumes sugar 3 to 4 times the safe limit every day for years.

And it gets worse. This self-destructive lifestyle isn't just limited to adults—it's being normalized in children. Parents feed their kids Red 40-laced snacks, sugar-loaded fruit juices, and seed oil-drenched processed foods as early as three years old. By the time they hit adolescence, their bodies are already inflamed, insulin-resistant, and addicted to sugar.

For the first time in over two centuries, the current generation of children in America may have shorter lifespans than their parents. Think about that. We are witnessing an entire population's health deteriorate in real-time, and most people either don't know or don't care.

The truth is, at this point, they are not even killing you—you are killing yourself.

Your health is your responsibility. Take accountability.

The Truth About Seed Oils: The Silent Killer in Your Food

Seed oils—such as canola, soybean, corn, sunflower, safflower, grapeseed, and cottonseed oil—are often marketed as "heart-healthy" alternatives to traditional fats. But the truth is, these industrial oils are highly processed, unstable, and toxic to the human body. They are cheap, chemically refined, and found in nearly every processed food, from cookies and cakes to salad dressings and fried foods. And they are killing people slowly but surely.

High in Inflammatory Omega-6 Fatty Acids

Your body needs a balance of omega-3 and omega-6 fatty acids, but seed oils overload the body with omega-6, leading to chronic inflammation. Inflammation is the root cause of heart disease, obesity, autoimmune disorders, and even cancer.

Linked to Hormonal Imbalances & Metabolic Disorders

The polyunsaturated fats (PUFAs) in seed oils are highly unstable, oxidizing easily when exposed to heat. This creates toxic free radicals that damage cells, disrupt hormones, and interfere with metabolism. Seed oils have been linked to:

Estrogen dominance and testosterone suppression

Obesity and insulin resistance

Thyroid dysfunction

Damaging to the Heart, Despite Being Called "Heart-Healthy"

The idea that seed oils are better for your heart than saturated fats is a complete lie. The original studies claimed this was industry-funded and ignored the fact that traditional fats (butter, tallow, olive oil, and coconut oil) have been used for centuries without causing heart disease. Meanwhile, heart disease skyrocketed after the introduction of processed seed oils.

Found in Everything: Cookies, Cakes, Fried Foods, and Even Salads

Baked goods (cookies, cakes, muffins, crackers) use seed oils because they are cheap, but these oxidized fats cause digestive inflammation and gut issues.

Fried foods (French fries, fried chicken, chips) absorb massive amounts of oxidized seed oils, making them a direct cause of artery-clogging inflammation and weight gain.

Salads and dressings often contain soybean or canola oil, which cancels out any nutritional benefits of the vegetables.

Cheap, Processed, and Marketed to Keep You Sick

Seed oils are cheap to produce, making them the go-to choice for food manufacturers and restaurants.

They replace high-quality fats like cold-pressed extra virgin olive oil, grass-fed butter, and coconut oil because they maximize profit at the expense of your health.

Most people, even maybe Google, will treat this as misinformation, but you don't want to trust these people, the ones making billions by lying to you,

causing you to eat the things you shouldn't eat, giving diseases you were never supposed to have in the first place. This proves these people's maliciousness; they lie to your face with no shame, no guilt.

That's exactly the problem—**mainstream narratives protect industries.** The food industry and its so-called "health experts" will always push **cheap, profitable, and mass-produced garbage** over the truth.

In the same way, they demonized **natural animal fats like butter and lard** while promoting **processed margarine and seed oils**, which turned out to be far worse.

You'll see why they defend seed oils when you follow the money. These oils are **a billion-dollar industry**, used in everything from packaged foods to fast food chains.

If people suddenly realized how toxic they are, **entire markets would collapse**—from the processed food industry to Big Pharma, which profits from the chronic diseases they cause.

Lies like this are why **obesity, diabetes, and cancer are skyrocketing.** It's why kids today are being raised on **chemical-laden, ultra-processed, inflammatory garbage** instead of real food. **Most people don't even question it.**

And some of these sheep even defend the ones who lie to us in order to make us sick. It's an evil world we live in.

The Long-Term Damage of Consuming Seed Oils

Regular consumption of seed oils has been linked to:

Obesity & metabolic syndrome

Alzheimer's & cognitive decline

Cancer cell growth due to oxidative stress

Heart disease & clogged arteries

Liver damage & fatty liver disease

What to Use Instead

Instead of toxic, cheap, and inflammatory seed oils, use:

Grass-fed butter & ghee (rich in vitamins and healthy fats)

Coconut oil (stable, antimicrobial, and great for high-heat cooking)

Beef tallow & lard (traditional fats that were unfairly demonized)

The Bottom Line: Avoid Seed Oils at All Costs

Seed oils are not food—they are industrial chemicals disguised as food. Avoid them entirely if you value your health, longevity, and hormone balance. These oils were introduced as a cheap alternative, but they come with a devastating cost to your body and long-term well-being. Stick to real, ancestral fats, and protect your health before it's too late.

Don't hit me with the *"it's too expensive to eat healthy."* You best believe it: **no amount of money can overvalue your health.**

Eat HEAL-THY

Remember

Nutrients, **Not Junk.**

Why would anyone eat something called "Junk" ?

Speaking of junk, let's talk about food dyes and artificial flavors.

Artificial flavors and food dyes are not just harmless additives—they are chemical cocktails designed to make processed foods more addictive while wreaking havoc on the body.

Many of these artificial ingredients, such as **Red 40, Yellow 5, and Blue 1,** have been linked to hyperactivity, mood disorders, and behavioral problems in children.

Studies suggest that these chemicals can trigger irritability, attention issues, and impulsivity, which are often misdiagnosed as ADHD.

Attention-deficit/hyperactivity disorder

Instead of addressing the real issue—diet—parents are pushed toward pharmaceutical solutions like ADHD medications, which generate billions for the drug industry.

Beyond behavior, artificial dyes and flavors have been linked to hormone disruption, allergic reactions, and even cancer in animal studies.

Countries like Europe have banned or required warning labels on certain dyes, yet in the U.S. and Canada, they are still being aggressively marketed to children through cereals, candies, and snacks.

These chemicals have zero nutritional value and serve only one purpose: to make processed junk look and taste more appealing while keeping consumers hooked.

The food industry profits off addiction, and Big Pharma profits off the health consequences. Meanwhile, the cycle of poor health, misdiagnosis, and medication dependency continues.

The ADHD medication industry is a multi-billion-dollar business driven by rising diagnosis rates, particularly among adults. In 2023, the global ADHD market was valued at $14.3 billion, with projections indicating continued growth.

Major pharmaceutical companies generate enormous profits from these drugs—Shire's Vyvanse alone made $1.4 billion in one year, while Eli Lilly's Strattera earned $579 million.

Between April 2020 and March 2022, new ADHD prescriptions increased by 32%, totaling nearly 1.4 million prescriptions.

As more people—especially children—are diagnosed with ADHD-like symptoms, often triggered by diet and environmental factors, the pharmaceutical industry continues to capitalize on medication as the primary "solution."

Instead of addressing underlying causes like artificial additives, sugar, and seed oils, the focus remains on prescription drugs, fueling an industry that thrives on dependency rather than long-term health solutions.

The Truth About Grains & Refined Carbohydrates

For centuries, grains were a staple in many traditional diets, but modern wheat and refined carbohydrates are nothing like their ancestral counterparts.

Today's wheat is heavily processed, stripped of nutrients, and loaded with glyphosate (a harmful pesticide).

The result? A hyper-processed, nutrient-deficient product that spikes blood sugar levels causes inflammation and contributes to metabolic disorders.

Gluten, found in most grains, has been linked to leaky gut syndrome, autoimmune diseases, and cognitive decline. It can cause digestive distress, bloating, and fatigue, even in people without celiac disease.

Worse, refined carbs like white bread, pasta, and pastries turn into sugar almost instantly in the body, leading to insulin resistance, obesity, and diabetes. The food industry promotes grains as "heart-healthy," but in reality, they are a key driver of inflammation, fat gain, and chronic disease.

Many people believe switching to a gluten-free diet automatically means eating healthier. However, most gluten-free processed foods are just as bad—if not worse—than their regular counterparts. When food companies remove gluten, they replace it with highly refined, inflammatory ingredients like:

Corn starch – High-glycemic filler that spikes blood sugar as fast as white flour.

Rice flour – Heavily processed, nutrient-poor, and high in arsenic.

Seed oils (canola, sunflower, soybean oil) – Cheap, toxic fats that cause inflammation.

Added sugars – Used to make gluten-free products taste better, often leading to higher sugar content than regular baked goods.

Gums & fillers (xanthan gum, guar gum, tapioca starch) – Used to mimic the texture of gluten but can cause bloating, digestive distress, and gut irritation.

While these products might be gluten-free, they are far from healthy. Many people who adopt gluten-free diets without proper knowledge still suffer from bloating, insulin resistance, inflammation, and weight gain because they consume processed alternatives instead of truly nutrient-dense foods.

The Solution: Ditch Processed Carbs & Choose Real, Nutrient-Dense Alternatives

Instead of replacing one processed food with another, focus on whole, real foods that nourish your body and avoid blood sugar spikes. Here's how:

Replace Refined Carbs & Flour with Nutrient-Dense Options

Instead of relying on processed gluten-free bread, crackers, and pastries, choose:

Sourdough bread (properly fermented, easier to digest, lower in gluten)

Almond flour or coconut flour (low-carb, fiber-rich alternatives for baking)

Cassava flour (gluten-free, minimally processed, better than corn or rice flour)

Sprouted grains (if tolerated, these are easier to digest and have better nutrient absorption)

You can even make your own pasta if you have good flour. Flour, eggs, olive oil, and salt.

Opt for Whole, Fiber-Rich Carbohydrates

Instead of processed gluten-free snacks, go for:

Sweet potatoes (rich in fiber, vitamins, and slower-digesting carbs)

Quinoa (a complete protein and a better alternative to refined rice)

Squash, pumpkin, or plantains (nutrient-dense, gut-friendly carbs)

Wild rice (lower in arsenic, richer in minerals than white rice)

Prioritize Protein & Healthy Fats Over Empty Carbs

Instead of making gluten-free processed foods the focus, build meals around protein and healthy fats, such as:

Grass-fed beef, wild-caught fish, pastured eggs (protein-rich and full of essential nutrients)

Avocados, olive oil, grass-fed butter (anti-inflammatory, heart-healthy fats)

Bone broth and organ meats (restore gut health and nutrient deficiencies)

The Bottom Line: Gluten-Free Doesn't Always Mean Healthy

The gluten-free industry is a multi-billion-dollar business, capitalizing on the idea that "gluten-free" = healthy. In reality, most gluten-free products are just as processed, sugar-laden, and inflammatory as regular junk food.

Instead of falling for the marketing, focus on whole, unprocessed, nutrient-dense foods that naturally support digestion, metabolism, and long-term health. It's just like the *"no added sugar"* label. A bait.

The Dangers of Overeating & Constant Snacking

One of the biggest nutritional myths is that you must eat every 2-3 hours to "boost metabolism." In reality, constantly eating keeps insulin elevated, preventing the body from burning fat.

The human body was designed to go through periods of eating and fasting, not to be constantly fed. The rise of hyper-palatable processed snacks has created a cycle of food addiction, cravings, and mindless eating.

Instead of listening to hunger cues, people eat out of boredom, habit, or emotional triggers, leading to weight gain, sluggish digestion, and metabolic dysfunction.

Your body releases insulin to store glucose every time you eat, especially carbs and processed foods. When insulin is constantly elevated due to frequent meals and snacks, your cells become resistant to it, leading to:

Higher fat storage (especially belly fat)

Increased risk of Type 2 diabetes

Hunger and cravings despite eating more

Energy crashes and brain fog

People think that eating frequently gives them energy, but in reality, it spikes and crashes blood sugar levels, leaving them feeling sluggish and constantly craving more food.

Digestion Needs Breaks – Overeating Wrecks the Gut

Your digestive system is not meant to be constantly working. When you eat all day, your gut never has time to process and clear food fully. This leads to:

Bloating, indigestion, and acid reflux

Leaky gut syndrome (where undigested food particles enter the bloodstream, triggering inflammation)

IBS and poor gut microbiome health

Fasting allows the gut to reset, repair, and reduce inflammation. When you constantly feed it junk, you overwhelm the system, leading to digestive dysfunction.

Overeating Ages You Faster

Constant eating activates mTOR, a cellular pathway that promotes growth and aging. While mTOR is essential for muscle building, overactivation through overeating accelerates aging and increases the risk of diseases like cancer.

On the other hand, fasting activates autophagy—the body's way of cleaning out damaged cells, reducing inflammation, and slowing aging. By eating less often and avoiding unnecessary snacking, you give your body a chance to repair itself instead of being stuck in digestion mode.

The Food Industry Promotes Snacking for Profits, Not Health

Think about it—who benefits when you eat six meals a day? The food industry, not you.

Snack companies push "healthy" granola bars, protein shakes, and small meals, tricking people into thinking they need constant fuel.

The truth? Ancient civilizations didn't eat every few hours, and they weren't weak or dying of malnutrition.

The rise of processed snacks perfectly aligns with the rise of obesity, diabetes, and metabolic syndrome.

The Solution: Eat Less Often, But More Nutrient-Dense Meals. Quality over quantity.

Instead of constantly grazing on junk, eat fewer but higher-quality meals:

Prioritize protein and healthy fats to keep you full longer.

Eat whole, unprocessed foods instead of ultra-processed snacks.

Try intermittent fasting (eating in a smaller window) to give your body time to burn fat and repair itself.

The Bottom Line: Less Eating = Better Health

The constant eating trend is a corporate-driven scam that keeps people overfed, sick, and dependent on food products. Humans are designed to eat, digest, and then stop eating for extended periods. Breaking free from frequent eating leads to fat loss, better digestion, sharper mental clarity, and a longer life.

Humans thrived on animal-based diets, whole foods, and natural fats for thousands of years. Yet, over the past century, these ancestral diets have been demonized while ultra-processed, low-fat, plant-based, and synthetic foods have been promoted as "healthier."

Butter, eggs, raw dairy, and organ meats—once considered nutritional powerhouses—were replaced with margarine, seed oils, refined carbs, starches, food dyes, and factory-farmed grains.

The result? Chronic disease, infertility, obesity, and mental health disorders skyrocketed. Traditional cultures that never suffered from modern diseases only started experiencing them when they adopted the Western diet.

Real food—meat, animal fats, seasonal fruits, and fermented foods—has been unfairly demonized in favor of cheap, highly profitable, lab-made substitutes. The truth? What worked for thousands of years doesn't suddenly become "unhealthy" because corporations say so.

The attack on meat conveniently ignores the real problem—factory-farmed meat. Unlike grass-fed, pasture-raised animals, factory-farmed meat comes from animals pumped with antibiotics, hormones and fed unnatural, grain-based diets.

This results in toxic, inflammation-causing meat that is then blamed for health issues. Similarly, farmed fish are raised in polluted environments, treated with dyes and chemicals, and fed processed pellets instead of natural diets.

When people claim that meat is bad for health, they are often referring to the industrial, low-quality version—not real, ethically raised meat.

The healthiest protein sources come from wild-caught fish, grass-fed beef, pasture-raised eggs, and organ meats, not chemically altered factory products. If you avoid high-quality animal foods, you're missing out on some of the most nutrient-dense foods on the planet.

The human body was never meant to be constantly fed. Fasting is one of the oldest, most effective health practices, yet modern society has made people believe they must eat every few hours.

When you fast, your body switches from burning glucose to burning fat, activates autophagy (cellular repair), reduces inflammation, and balances hormones. Studies show that fasting improves insulin sensitivity, supports brain function, and promotes longevity.

Despite this, mainstream nutritionists warn against fasting, claiming it's "dangerous"—when, in reality, nothing could be more natural.

Whether through intermittent fasting, one meal a day (OMAD), or extended fasts, allowing your body time to rest from digestion leads to higher energy, better focus, and improved metabolic health. Fasting isn't about starvation—it's healing.

WEIGHT LOSS

Why the "Calories In, Calories Out" Model is Flawed

One of the biggest lies in modern nutrition is that **weight loss is simply about eating fewer calories than you burn.** This outdated model ignores **hormonal balance, food quality, and metabolic health.**

The body does not process **100 calories of steak** the same way it does **100 calories of soda.** Nutrient-dense foods provide **satiety, muscle preservation, and metabolic benefits,** while processed junk disrupts hormones and increases cravings. Insulin, not just calories, plays a major role in **fat storage and hunger regulation.**

Highly processed foods **spike insulin, leading to energy crashes and fat accumulation,** while protein and healthy fats stabilize blood sugar and **support muscle growth.**

If calories were the only thing that mattered, then people eating the same number of calories in junk food and whole foods would have the same health outcomes—but they don't.

For decades, people have been told that weight loss is just about "calories in, calories out" (CICO)—that if you eat fewer calories than you burn, you'll lose weight.

While this model isn't completely false, it ignores how different foods, hormones, and metabolic processes affect fat loss. The body is not a simple calculator—it's a complex system regulated by insulin, hormones, and energy balance.

You Don't Have to Count Calories to Lose Weight

Weight loss isn't just about eating less—it's about eating right. When you eat real, whole foods, your body naturally regulates hunger, metabolism, and fat-burning. The reason most people fail on low-calorie diets is because they still eat processed junk, keeping them hungry, inflamed, and insulin resistant. Instead of obsessing over numbers, focus on:

Cutting out sugar, refined carbs, and seed oils

Prioritizing nutrient-dense foods like meat, eggs, and healthy fats

Eating fewer but higher-quality meals

Fasting regularly to reset metabolism

When you do this, your body will naturally adjust food intake and start burning stored fat for energy, without needing to micromanage every calorie.

Let Your Body Burn Fat Through Fasting & Exercise

One of the biggest mistakes people make is eating too frequently. When you eat all day long—especially carbs—you constantly spike insulin, which tells your body to store fat instead of burning it. The key to effective fat loss is to:

Fast regularly (e.g., intermittent fasting, OMAD, 24-hour fasts)
Exercise while fasting to force the body to burn stored fat
Eat whole, unprocessed foods to prevent insulin spikes

Fasting causes your body to enter a state where it burns stored fat instead of constantly processing new food.

Exercising While Fasting – The Best Weight Loss Hack

Many people believe you must eat before a workout to have energy. This is a myth. When fasting, your body switches to using fat for fuel, making workouts even more effective.

Fasted exercise boosts fat-burning hormones like adrenaline and norepinephrine.
It improves insulin sensitivity, making it easier to lose weight.
It doesn't harm muscle mass unless you fast for extremely long periods.
You'll feel strong and energized as long as you stay hydrated and aren't too deep into a fast.

One of the best times to work out while fasting is the morning after an overnight fast (perfect for weight loss). 4-6 hours into a fast, before breaking it with a protein-rich meal

The Truth About Jump Rope – Why It's a Fat-Burning Machine

Jumping rope is one of the most underrated but effective weight-loss workouts. Here's why:

Burns more calories per minute than running (a 10-minute jump rope session can burn the same as a 30-minute jog) Full-body workout – engages legs, core, shoulders, and arms Boosts cardiovascular endurance – great for heart health and stamina Improves coordination and agility – used by boxers and elite athletes Low impact if done properly – easier on joints than running

If you combine jump rope with fasting, your body burns even more fat since it taps into stored energy reserves.

Why Sugar, Seed Oils, and Processed Foods Stop Fat Loss

You can work out daily, but if you're eating sugar, processed carbs, and seed oils, you may find yourself struggling to lose weight or wondering why you're constantly bloated. These foods:

Spike insulin, preventing fat-burning Cause inflammation, leading to bloating and water retention Mess with hunger hormones, making you crave more junk Get stored as fat quickly, especially in the belly

When you stop eating refined carbs, sugar, and processed junk, your body naturally shifts into a fat-burning state.

Stop Eating for Pleasure – Eat for Nourishment, Purpose Over Pleasure

Most people are addicted to food—they eat not because they're hungry but because they're bored, emotional, or craving sugar. This is why:

Fasting helps reset your hunger signals so you eat when truly needed.
Breaking a fast with real, whole foods (meat, eggs, healthy fats) fuels your body correctly.
Refueling with sugar or junk after fasting leads to fat gain because your body absorbs nutrients more efficiently post-fast (which is what most people do in the morning).

Fat Loss is a Lifestyle, Not Just a Diet

Losing weight isn't about starving yourself or tracking every calorie. It's about:
Eating real, unprocessed food
Fasting regularly to reset metabolism
Exercising in a fasted state for maximum fat burn
Ditching sugar, seed oils, and refined carbs permanently
Choosing workouts like jump rope for high-intensity fat loss

Fat loss happens naturally and effortlessly once you stop feeding your body junk and give it the right fuel. The human body isn't meant to be fat; it is meant to be athletic, strong, and resilient. Being fat may be normal, but never forget; in this world, normal doesn't mean good.

The Lies Are Everywhere, But So Is the Truth

Nearly everything we've been told about diet, nutrition, and health is a carefully crafted lie to benefit corporations, not people. The food industry creates sickness, Big Pharma profits from managing it, and mainstream nutrition "experts" reinforce the cycle.

The truth is simple:

Eat real, whole, unprocessed foods. Avoid toxic ingredients like seed oils, refined sugar, and artificial additives.

Use fasting and meal timing to optimize metabolism. Reject corporate food propaganda and return to ancestral wisdom.

Mastery

Easier said than done.

"Never put off until tomorrow what can be done today."

From Knowledge to Action

What good is all this knowledge if you don't apply it? You can start today. Change your life, change your future, change who you are.

There is no shortcut, no secret formula—the only way to reclaim your health and free yourself from the lies of the food industry is through pure discipline and willpower.

You either make the choice to prioritize your health or continue slowly destroying yourself. Most people know they are ruining their bodies, but they do nothing to change. That is the definition of failure.

Don't be like them.

Master Your Food Discipline with Fasting

Start with 12 hours a day, let your body adjust.

Gradually increase to 16, then 18, then 24 hours.

Push yourself to a full 48-hour fast—feel the reset, the clarity, the transformation.

Once ready, attempt a 24-hour dry fast.

Gain experience, push further, challenge yourself—maybe even a 48-hour dry fast.

Fasting is your greatest tool. It forces discipline, resets your metabolism, detoxes your system, and strengthens your mind.

When you relapse into bad habits, use fasting to purge the addiction. If you think your discipline is well-developed simply because you exercise a lot, try fasting. You're going to hit a wall.

Reset Your Body – Cut the Sugar, Cut the Processed Food

Never break your fast with junk—your body absorbs nutrients more efficiently post-fast.

Refuel with whole, natural foods—meat, eggs, avocado, real fats.

The moment you stop eating sugar and processed food, your body begins to heal.

If you relapse, don't dwell on failure—go on a fast to detox and start fresh.

This isn't a one-time thing—it's a way of life. Every time you step back, you push forward harder.

Educate Yourself & Teach Others

The more you learn about nutrition, fasting, and real health, the stronger you become.

Teach others—because explaining something forces you to understand it deeper.

The more knowledge you share, the harder it is to fall back into ignorance.

Your Future Self Will Thank You

It will be hard at first. Your mind will crave the dopamine hits of junk food, laziness, and instant gratification. But over time, your desires will change.

You won't crave sugar, processed food, or toxic junk—because you will no longer be an addict.

You won't seek comfort—you will seek growth.

You will choose nutrients over junk.

You will prefer actions over mere talk.

You will embrace exercise over laziness.

You will put purpose over pleasure.

Master your desires, or they will master you. It's easier said than done, but never put off until tomorrow what can be done today.

Health is Wealth.

Sayonara

Until Next Time.

If you enjoyed this book, please leave a review on Amazon and don't hesitate to share it with your surroundings. It may seem short but it's enough. Just like your meals should be, quality over quantity.

Message me at mrlemy4@gmail.com , if you please.

Remember, this book isn't just a read, it's a study. If you study in depth every aspect of this book, it'll be worth your while. Your knowledge levels will skyrocket, and your mind won't be blinded by the illusions of this world. Start Today.

If you liked this book and long for more, please send me an email, I will respond and be encouraged to put out more.

Until Next Time,

Take Care.

www.ingramcontent.com/pod-product-compliance
Lightning Source LLC
Chambersburg PA
CBHW050215270326
41914CB00003BA/424